THE NATURAL WAY SERIES

Increasing numbers of people worldwide are falling victim to illnesses which modern medicine, for all its technical advances, seems often powerless to prevent – and sometimes actually causes. To help with these so-called 'diseases of civilization' more and more people are turning to 'natural' medicine for an answer. The *Natural Way* series aims to offer clear, practical and reliable guidance to the safest, gentlest and most effective treatments available – and so to give sufferers and their families the information they need to make their own choices about the most suitable treatments.

Other titles in the Natural Way *series*

Allergies
Arthritis & Rheumatism
Asthma
Cancer
Chronic Fatigue Syndrome
Colds & Flu
Cystitis
Diabetes
Eczema
Heart Disease
HIV & Aids
Infertility
Irritable Bowel Syndrome
Migraine
Multiple Sclerosis
Premenstrual Syndrome
Psoriasis

The Natural Way

Back Pain

Helena Bridge

Series medical consultants
Dr Peter Albright MD (USA)
& Dr David Peters MD (UK)

Approved by the
AMERICAN HOLISTIC MEDICAL ASSOCIATION
& BRITISH HOLISTIC MEDICAL ASSOCIATION

E L E M E N T

Shaftesbury, Dorset ● Rockport, Massachusetts
Melbourne, Victoria

© Element Books Limited 1995
Text © Helena Bridge 1995

First published in the UK in 1995 by
Element Books Limited
Shaftesbury, Dorset SP7 8BP

Published in the USA in 1995 by
Element Books, Inc.
PO Box 830, Rockport, MA 01966

Published in Australia in 1995 by
Element Books
and distributed by
Penguin Books Australia Limited
487 Maroondah Highway, Ringwood, Victoria 3134

Reprinted 1995
Reissued 1998

Cover design by Slatter-Anderson
Designed and typeset by Linda Reed and Joss Nizan
Printed and bound in Great Britain

British Library Cataloguing in Publication

Library of Congress Cataloging in Publication Data
Bridge, Helena.
The natural way with back pain/Helena Bridge
p. cm. --(The Natural way series)
Includes bibliographical references and index.
ISBN 1-85230-581-9
1. Backache–Alternative treatment. 2. Naturopathy. I. Title.
II. Series.
RD771.B217B75 1995
617.5'64--dc20 94-47047
CIP

ISBN 1 85230 581 9

Contents

List of illustrations   vi
Acknowledgements   viii
Introduction   1

Chapter 1   **What is back pain?**   3
Chapter 2   **All about your back**   10
Chapter 3   **Causes and risk factors
             in back pain**   20
Chapter 4   **How to help yourself**   44
Chapter 5   **Conventional treatments
             and procedures**   63
Chapter 6   **The natural therapies
             and back pain**   81
Chapter 7   **Treating your body**   89
Chapter 8   **Treating your mind
             and emotions**   100
Chapter 9   **'Energy' therapies that can help
             back pain**   112
Chapter 10   **How to find and choose a
             natural therapist**   126

Glossary   141
Appendix A **Useful organizations**   142
Appendix B **Useful further reading**   146
Index   147

List of Illustrations

Figure 1	The spine, showing four curves	11
Figure 2	The bones, joints and nerves of the spine	12
Figure 3	How joints move	16
Figure 4	Referred pain 'maps'	23
Figure 5	Abdominal exercises	59–60
Figure 6	An Alexander Technique relaxation exercise	91
Figure 7	'The Cat' yoga exercise for backs	98
Figure 8	Acupuncture 'energy' meridians and main points	115
Figure 9	Reflexology zones on the right foot	123

For Robert

Acknowledgements

Many people helped me write this book but special thanks go to my friend, author Angela Smyth, for providing the impetus, to the series editor Richard Thomas for his vision and good-natured patience, and to Julia McCutchen of Element Books for her moral support. For the prompt supply of information I am indebted to the Research Council for Complementary Medicine, the UK National Back Pain Association, the British Chiropractic Association, the Osteopathic Information Service and Penny Crowther of Cantassium Ltd. To numerous therapists and practitioners, especially Valerie Brown, P. J. Cousin, Ian Lambert and Dr David Owen, go my grateful thanks for help and suggestions. Finally, heartfelt thanks to Andrew Bryant and Lizzie Neil for looking after my patients while I finished work on the book.

Introduction

Back pain may be a joke to many but to those who suffer it is far from funny. In extreme cases it can cause excruciating pain as well as be severely disabling. Sufferers may not be able to walk let alone work.

What is not often understood by those who laugh is that back pain can happen to almost anyone at any time. If it has not yet happened to you the chances are it will! Back pain affects almost everyone at some point in their life and most of us know at least someone who is affected.

The scale of the problem is actually enormous. In most Western countries, back pain is the single biggest cause of absence from work after flu. The statistics tell the staggering story.

- More than 90 million working days are lost in the UK alone from long-term absence (that is, people being off work for over a month), and the number is rising dramatically every year.
- Every year in the USA 12 million Americans see their doctor about some new back problem.
- 100 million visits a year in the USA are made to chiropractors (specialists in back pain).

And these figures show only the tip of the iceberg. They do not include short-term absences, self-employed people, married women, widows, pensioners and most government employees. They also leave out the many head, neck, arm and leg pains which can come with back problems. So the true picture really is of staggering proportions – and getting worse.

But what is worse still is the number of people who, lacking faith in modern drugs and afraid of surgery, suffer in silence quite needlessly. Back pain is a serious and disabling condition but it can be cured without either drugs or surgery. There are a number of gentler and safer options you can try.

This book aims to introduce you to those gentler, safer and, usually, highly effective options. In particular it will:

- help you understand your back and why it sometimes hurts
- help you help your own back, whether you are in pain or not
- lead you through conventional methods of treating back pain
- introduce you to the wide range of gentler options, including natural therapies with a good track record of helping back pain
- help you decide whether natural therapy might be right for you
- help you find the right natural therapist

So whether this is your first encounter with back pain, whether you are someone who has suffered for so long you feel nothing can be done and you must simply 'live with it', or whether you have not yet had a problem but are afraid you might, this book is your guide to a new back – a healthy back.

Helena Bridge

CHAPTER 1

What is back pain?

How it happens and who it affects

Back pain can come in any area of the back, from the top of the neck to the tailbone. The most common type is pain in the lower part of the back. Low back pain, as it is known, is the most common reason for time lost at work. But back pain can come in many other forms too.

The different types of back pain

The following are the main types of back pain. (Medical names are in italics and are explained more fully in Chapter 2.)

Low back pain

Better known as *lumbago*, this is normally an aching discomfort at waist level. It can include pain around to one side or other, or both. If the pain is lower down, where the spine joins the buttock area, it is called *lumbosacral pain*. This can extend downwards and out into the buttock muscles which often feel 'bruised'.

In severe cases, pain down the leg comes on with (and sometimes without) low back pain. This is widely known as *sciatica*, even though it may be nothing to do with the sciatic nerve itself. It can go right down the back or side of the leg into the foot. Putting weight on that leg, or even just putting your foot to the floor, might be impossible, and putting on clothes becomes a circus act!

Most low back pain generally comes on after lifting or twisting, either suddenly or over a period of time. It is often made worse by standing, loafing about, sitting or bending forwards.

The lower back area is the one most commonly affected by *disc* problems, followed by the neck area. However, they rarely occur in the *thoracic* spine except as a result of serious accidents. Discs are discussed in more detail later.

Neck pain

This is the next most common after low back pain. It can be anything from a tired ache to a complete 'jam-up', allowing little movement in any direction. Neck problems usually result from a combination of tension and misuse. Most of us carry our heads too far forwards, and this puts too much strain on the delicate tissues at the back which hold our heads up. Neck problems often extend upwards causing headaches, dizziness, eye pains, migraines and nausea. Less commonly, neck trouble can cause ear, jaw or dental pains.

Thoracic pain

This is back pain anywhere from the base of the neck to the top of the waist – that is, at any level of the chest. This part of the spine is different because it has ribs attached to it. Ribs act as stabilizers for the spine, but there are also more joints and muscles to go wrong in this area.

Thoracic back pain can be very sharp, especially if one of the ribs has been wrenched. The pain may shoot right around to the front. Thoracic pain can also be linked to the way the shoulder-blades are moving against the back. If there are problems here the pain can be very wearing, especially if you work with your arms out-stretched on a conveyor belt or at a keyboard.

General back pain

Although we can divide back pain into different areas many people don't fall into these neat groups. Lots of people suffer from all of them. Not only that, but the range of their symptoms is much wider and more varied than those described above. The pain 'menu' of the human back includes, in order of how commonly the symptoms occur:

- dull aches which may throb, wake you up at night or simply wear you down
- stiffness on moving in one or more directions (these can make you feel very old)
- pain on moving towards a painful 'barrier' (this can be very sharp, and may also apply to several directions of movement at once)
- sharp pains, either stabbing or shooting, which can be severe enough to make you catch your breath
- a feeling of 'deadness', 'heaviness', 'numbness' or 'pins and needles', rather like a limb 'going to sleep' (this is where the circulation is likely to be impaired or a nerve compressed)
- an unpleasant electrical-type 'tingling' sensation (which doctors call *paraesthesia*) where a nerve may be compressed or starved of its blood supply
- true 'numbness' (or *anaesthesia*) where there is actual loss of skin sensation, which can be tested
- supersensitive skin which feels as though it has been rubbed with sandpaper (called *hyperaesthesia*)

The list above outlines common symptoms but if yours are different don't worry. Everyone's symptoms vary and are unique to them at that moment. What is much more important is to know why all this happens in the first place.

What can lead to back pain

Just as the symptoms of back pain are many, the causes are too. In order of seriousness they boil down to three main things (terms in *italics* are explained more fully in the next chapter):

- tissues held tight under strain
- tissue damage
- disease

(*Tissues* mean any group of cells in the body with the same structure and function. This can mean anything from *bone*, *muscle* or *cartilage*, to *blood vessels*, *nerves* and so on.)

Tissues held tight under strain covers situations like muscles in *spasm*, compressed nerves, bulging *discs* and twisted joints, for example. The many strained postures we adopt to compensate for pain and loss of movement also come under this heading. Pain in all these cases is caused by a torrent of signals from the stretched or squashed tissues.

Actual *tissue damage* applies to more dramatic events like broken bones, *stress fractures*, torn *ligaments* and muscles, worn and damaged cartilage, *disc herniation*, and torn nerves. One of the main sources of pain in these examples is *inflammation*, the body's first response to tissue damage. Inflammation brings local heat, swelling and chemical irritation from the waste products of the healing process. Our bodies are very neatly packed so inflamed swellings hurt.

Disease can exist in the tissues of the spine or its attachments (bones, muscles, discs or ligaments) or anywhere else in the body. Either way, back pain is likely to be a feature in many instances. Pain from disease can be through swelling from infections or tumours, irritation by body poisons and nervous irritation from the site of disease to the spinal cord.

Back pain, then, has many causes. But 'backbone pain', even if the pain is severe, is rarely caused by the backbone itself any more than it is caused by disease. The most common causes *are* mechanical, but from a variety of sources. And they don't strike randomly like lightning, they 'accumulate'. Our backs are a living diary of how we have used and misused them.

Sooner or later the effects of dozens of falls, accidents, emotional shocks, plus years of bad diet and bad posture, all add up to back pain. For most people it is sooner rather than later. Let's look at which groups of people get back pain and when.

Who is most affected

Although accidents account for many back injuries most, according to the British National Back Pain Association, occur when people repeat movements that have previously been no problem. Back pain, it reports, occurs most of all in the 16–44 age group. People at highest risk are those who have already had a back problem – something like 80 per cent suffer a recurrence. In the end, though, it seems that everyone is at risk, including:

- children and teenagers – mostly from accidents but also through slouching at school, carrying heavy books, and either lack of exercise or overtraining and injuring themselves at sport (very young children can sometimes also suffer back pain from unresolved birth strains)

- adults 'in their prime' – from a string of reasons covering home, work and play. The following are among the most common causes of adult back pain:

At home Lifting children or furniture, using incorrect movements to do the ironing, bed-making, vacuuming, gardening, cleaning in general and cleaning the bath in particular, driving a car – the list is endless.

At sports General lack of exercise followed by vigorous sport, often without enough of a warm-up period.

At work There were 33,000 back *accidents* in the UK in 1992–3, and 500,000 work-related back conditions (not diseases).

Listed below are adults who are particularly vulnerable to back problems.

- Nurses are at very high risk, with nearly a tenth of the nursing work force having back injuries at any one time. In the UK, for example, the total cost of nurse absence and replacement due to back pain is now running at £120 million a year.

- Computer screen operators – about eight out of ten operators of VDUs will suffer back pain.

- Office workers and other sedentary (seated) workers get just as much back pain as manual workers.

- People who drive for a living are three times more likely to suffer than those whose work does not involve driving.

- Old people – many elderly people's spines are worn from a lifetime of work, gravity, 'knocks and shocks' and bad habits. Arthritic knees and hips can also contribute to the back pain figures, by forcing elderly backs into bad postures.

- Heavy smokers whose circulation has been affected by heavy and long-term smoking are generally less able to recover from back injuries.

- Those who persistently abuse drugs and other addictive substances can have unhealthy tissues, prone to injury and slow to heal.

Summary

It is clear that back pain is caused by many different factors and affects just about everyone. But perhaps the most significant fact is that once you start to suffer you are likely to go on suffering unless you do something about it. And you *can* do something about it. The first stage in doing something is to learn a little more about your back and how it works.

CHAPTER 2

All about your back

What it is and how it works

Apart from keeping us upright, our back serves two main purposes: it allows us to move freely and it protects our spinal cord. Movement keeps us healthy, while protection is essential for the spinal cord because it is the vital but delicate extension of the brain which spreads movement and sensations to every part of our body.

There is a close connection between our mind and our body and this is particularly so in our back, and specifically in our spine. In this way our backs become a playground for our feelings. So our backs are affected by everything we do, whether for good or bad. This means that there are not only many causes of back pain but many ways of relieving it too.

But the first step in any treatment is understanding a bit about how the back functions in the way it does, how it connects to the rest of our body and what it needs to stay fit and healthy.

The spine

As figure 1 shows, our spines consist of a column of 24 individual bones called *vertebrae*, five fused vertebrae called sacrum, and the four fused bones of the coccyx. Between each vertebra and the next is a springy shock-absorbing disc (or *intervertebral disc* to give it its full name). Together the vertebrae and discs make up the *vertebral column* with seven cervical, twelve thoracic and five lumbar vertebrae. The spine has four curves (see below).

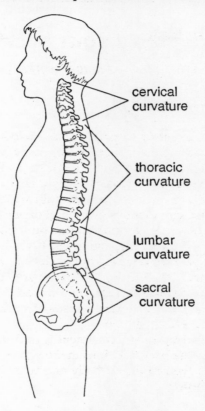

Fig 1. The spine, showing four curves

Running down the full length of this column is a series of bony arches forming a tunnel. These arches are attached, rather like drawer-handles, to the back of each vertebra. Each 'drawer-handle', or *vertebral arch*, has a 'spine' sticking out of the back of it and these are the 'knobbly bits' we can feel all down our backs (*see figure 2*).

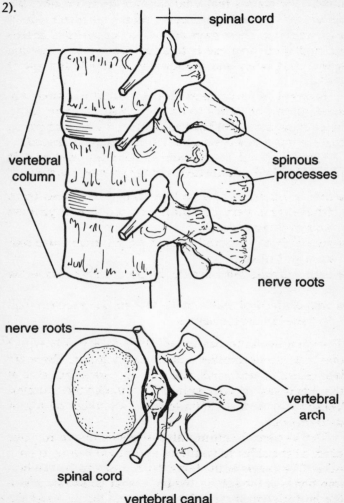

Fig 2. Bones, joints and nerves of the spine

The tunnel of vertebral arches, lined and covered by long bands of tough elastic tissue, is called the *vertebral canal*. This houses that vital communication centre, the *spinal cord*. The only gaps in the tunnel are either side of each vertebra. These gaps are called *intervertebral foramina*, and their purpose is to allow nerves to leave the spinal cord safely and comfortably to supply the rest of the body.

Each spinal nerve takes care of a handful of body tissues, giving branches to areas of bone, muscle, joint, inner organ and skin. Most areas share a nerve supply so that there is a 'reserve circuit' if one nerve is damaged.

For the spinal nerve roots to have a pain-free exit from the spinal column each gap (or *foramen*) must be:

- free of outcrops of vertebral bone jutting into them (these form very commonly in old age, a process known as *spondylosis*)
- free of bulky scarred ligaments, joint capsules and damaged discs
- well supplied with healthy blood vessels to serve the nerve roots
- well drained of waste fluids that could otherwise collect and irritate the nerves

The spinal column has some 150 *joints* – points where one bone meets another and levers against it. There are two chains of *facet joints*, one running down each side of the 'knobbles' of your spine, deep under the muscles. These allow each vertebra to move smoothly on top of its neighbour.

The vertebral column also attaches above to your head, at the sides to your ribs and down below to your *pelvis*. The pelvis is the bony 'basin' formed by the bottom bones of the spine – the big triangular *sacrum* above the buttock-crease, and the tailbone or *coccyx* – and the two big 'hip bones', called the *innominate bones*.

These joints – where the spine meets the head, ribs and pelvis – are key points for back injuries caused by misuse. Each joint of the spine can only take a certain amount of strain and movement, and overloading these important areas is common.

The importance of the discs

Discs (*see figure 2*) are vital to the spinal column – without them you would look like you'd swallowed an umbrella. You'd be straight and stiff. The discs attach firmly above and below to the flat surfaces of the vertebrae. They keep our spines flexible and work as shock-absorbers for all spinal movements.

Discs can do these things because of their structure, which gives both strength and flexibility. The strength comes from the *annulus fibrosus*, an outer wall made of many concentric rings of fibres, each layer running in a slightly different direction. This way they stay strong whichever way we stretch them. The flexibility comes from their soft centre, the *nucleus pulposus*, that consists of a thick gel held between the vertebrae under high pressure.

How discs work

Gravity and compression squeezes fluid from the soft-centred nucleus into the linking vertebrae, which act as bony sponges. It is only when we lie down and rest that this effect is reversed – the fluid refills the disc which swells up to become more springy again. This is why people are actually taller in the mornings than in the evenings.

Discs dry out as the years go by, as all body tissues do. The disc centres lose some of their 'juiciness' and their walls harden. The bad news about this is that our spines become stiffer with old age. But the good news is that the risk of disc problems reduces as a result.

How the spine got its curves

Seen from the side, the spine of a newborn baby looks like a letter C. Once the baby can hold its head up its neck muscles begin to pull its *cervical spine* (the neck portion) into the first of two forward curves. This is called the *cervical lordosis*. Once the baby learns to sit up the muscles of the lower back pull it forwards in the waist area, too, to form the *lumbar lordosis*.

The area curving backwards between the two lordoses of the spine is at chest level, and is called the *thoracic kyphosis*. This backward direction is matched at both ends of the spine by the curves of the back of the head and the pelvis.

From head to tail, then, this wavey line of bones and joints (*see figure 1*) is protecting its precious contents by being adapted to absorb mechanical shocks, stresses and strains, some quite severe, for many years.

How the back moves

Besides protecting the spinal cord, one of the main functions of the back is to move. Movement is allowed at the facet joints, discs and ribs, and is limited by muscles and *ligaments* – tough bands of fibrous, slightly elastic tissue which act like 'sticky-tape' across the joints.

If bone were just to rub against bone inside the joints a fire would eventually start. Painful heat and friction are prevented in healthy joints by the bones being tightly covered with a smooth white layer of *hyaline cartilage*. The bones are held together in a sealed unit by a tough *joint capsule*. This has a velvety lining layer called *synovial membrane* which constantly oozes and reabsorbs an oily liquid called *synovial fluid*. There are no blood vessels between the joint surfaces as these would be damaged by weight and friction. It is the synovial fluid

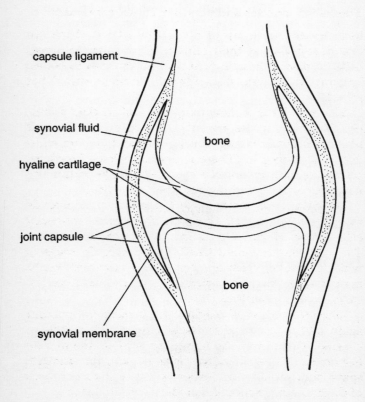

capsule ligament

synovial fluid

hyaline cartilage

joint capsule

synovial membrane

bone

bone

Fig 3. How joints move

which nourishes and lubricates these surfaces, making them as slippery as ice sliding on ice (*see figure 3*).

Joints, then, are well designed for movement but they need something to do the actual moving. This is where the *muscles* come in.

The role of muscles and nerves in spinal movement

Muscles are made up of many fine fibres which are drawn together at their ends to form tougher bands called *tendons*. These in turn connect muscles to bones, knitting firmly into the 'skin' of the bone, called the *periosteum*.

The muscles that move bones are called *skeletal muscles*. Skeletal muscles are either able to contract at will like the biceps or control fine balance and posture without us knowing it. (There is another type of muscles called *involuntary muscles* and these make automatic movements like breathing and goose pimples.)

To make them move skeletal muscles need signals from the *motor nerves*. These are fine chains of special cells linking the brain to the muscles via the spinal cord. The desire to move is turned into an electrical signal, which flits along from one nerve cell to the next, jumping across the gaps (or *synapses*) using chemical 'ferries' called *neurotransmitters*.

Once the message reaches the muscle the current again sets off chemical reactions, causing the muscle to shorten. This moves the bones at the joints the muscle lies across. The well-known *biceps* muscle, for example, spans both shoulder and elbow joints so it acts on both of them to bring a spoonful of food to your mouth.

The importance of blood and lymph

All the structures mentioned so far depend on blood to maintain them. This is pumped down ever smaller arteries until it reaches the tiny *capillaries*, blood vessels whose walls are only one cell thick and which each supply a small group of cells.

Here, at tissue level, dissolved oxygen and food crosses into the cells. 'Used blood' is then carried back to the lungs to pick up more oxygen from the air we breathe. Food substances in the bloodstream are mixed with this and pumped back out to the tissues by the heart.

All cells produce a clear waste fluid called *lymph*. This is squeezed out into little tubes called *lymphatic vessels* which form a network running parallel to the veins.

Lymph fluid has to pass through various important filtering stations along its way to the heart and then return to the circulation. These filtering stations lie in body creases like the armpits and groin, and are commonly called 'glands'. They are, in fact, correctly called lymph *nodes*, and their purpose is to filter all lymph fluid and kill off any infected material using special immune cells produced within the nodes.

The importance of exercise

Unlike arteries, where blood is pushed along by the pumping action of the heart and arterial pulses, neither veins nor lymphatics possess any 'pump'. They get little help from the heart to return used blood and lymph to it for recycling. Instead they rely on exercise which causes contracting muscles surrounding the vessels to squeeze these fluids back (usually up) to the heart.

The health of the circulatory system therefore depends on us moving about freely – that is, by exercising. In turn our ability to exercise depends on us having a healthily moving spine. In other words the circulation of body fluids and the health of the human back are crucial and interdependent.

The importance of connective tissue

One important ingredient is missing from this explanation so far: *connective tissue*. This tissue provides a universal 'sleeve' for all the structures of the body, including the spine and all its attachments.

Connective tissue gets everywhere – every muscle, bone, nerve, blood and lymphatic vessel, every organ of the body, is covered in a close-fitting sheath of connective tissue.

It is actually specialized connective tissue that forms all the ligaments, the disc walls, joint capsules and tendons. In some places, notably in the lower half of the spine, broad sheets of connective tissue (called *fascia*) provide a fixing for the large muscles of the back and shoulders.

There are also whole sheets of fascia running between the muscle layers, serving as further stabilizers for the body. In addition they screen off whole sections of the body from each other, thus helping to prevent the spread of infection.

In common with almost all the structures described so far, connective tissue can be injured and is sensitive to pain.

Summary

So much for the mechanics then. But what *is* pain, and what sort of damage can cause back pain? What are its main triggers and what are the risk factors? In the next chapter we'll look in more detail at pain and its causes as well as what a health professional looks at when you turn up with back pain.

CHAPTER 3

Causes and risk factors in back pain

What they are and how they affect us

The health of the human back depends on a variety of factors but they all fall into three simple groupings: structural, nutritional and emotional.

'Structural factors' are those which affect the mechanics of the spinal 'building blocks', while 'nutritional' factors govern what goes into the making and mending of them. 'Emotional' factors affect the inner stresses we put on the structure.

The important point here is that back pain generally *does not come from mechanical strain alone*. Our backs express our health at all levels, and an emotional upset can send our backs into painful spasm as easily as heavy lifting can.

Also, if we did not eat well at an important stage of our growth, or during a period of emotional upheaval, this can make matters even worse, as our tissues will be more prone to injury and slower to heal.

Structure, nutrition and emotions, like a three-legged stool, are the three vital components of everyone's health. If any one is slightly out or deficient the stool is off-balance and could topple. So it is with your back.

Usually the immediate cause of back pain *is* mechanical – but a wise therapist would want to know a lot more about your lifestyle and background to discover if there are other contributing factors hidden away that made it easier or more likely for you to succumb.

They would want to know if you have been eating a proper balanced diet, for example, or if you have been under emotional pressures. Is there someone at work, perhaps, who 'won't get off your back'? Or are you 'carrying the world on your shoulders'?

Emotional pain can quite easily lead to physical pain as well as vice versa, and it is worth looking at pain more closely. What is it, and why do some people seem to feel it more than others? More to the point, what could have caused *your* back pain and is it serious?

What happens when we feel pain

It is important to realize that you only 'feel' pain once it is translated into a conscious feeling in your brain. Pain is not an event that happens in the painful tissue itself or in the nerves that carry the message. Pain is always 'in the mind', but this does not mean that it is imaginary. There is just no measurable event called pain that exists outside our minds.

As pain is impossible to measure it is not fair to judge someone's pain by how you think you would react in the same situation. By the same token we can improve our ability to cope with pain by changing our attitude towards it.

The positive role of pain

Pain is one of the main ways we have of protecting ourselves against damage because it discourages us from repeating the activity that aroused it. For pain to be a useful warning sign the nerves which signal it have to be just about everywhere: almost every tissue in the body has specialized pain-sensitive nerve endings called *pain receptors* (that is, they *receive* painful input).

What triggers pain?

The most obvious event that triggers pain is damage to body tissues. This is registered by the pain receptors (or *nociceptors*). Other types of nerve endings can signal pain too if pushed beyond their limits – for example, by:

● too much heat or cold
● too bright a light
● too loud a sound
● too much pressure (or *compression*)
● too little circulation
● too much swelling
● too much stretch

These widespread pain responses protect both our special senses (such as sight, hearing, smell, taste and touch), and our inner organs (for example the heart, lungs and digestive and sex organs).

Let's look now at how the inner organs register pain, and what this has to do with your back.

Different types of pain

A whole lot of symptoms were listed in Chapter 1 but there are still some further types of pain which complete the picture. For example, the inner organs are sensitive to stretch from within, to pressure from without and also to chemical irritation by bodily poisons (*toxins*).

When any set of nerve receptors in an organ is bombarded enough you will feel pain. You might not feel this near the organ itself. You might feel it in a completely separate region which happens to share the same nerve pathway to the brain. Such pain is called *referred pain*.

Many areas of referred pain are located in the back, which can make the job of deciding on the exact cause of pain more difficult (see 'Non-spinal causes', p. 31). Figure 4 shows the areas of the back where pain from various organs may be felt. This is why you should seek professional help if your back pain is not improving.

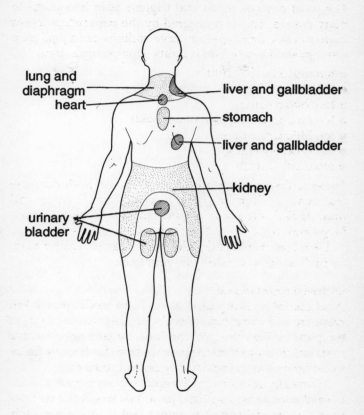

Fig 4. Referred pain 'maps'

Another term you might hear used to describe pain is *radiating pain*. This does exactly what it says – it radiates from the original source of pain along structures

connected to the local area of disease or *trauma* (injury).
It need not signify damage to a nerve itself, although the
term 'trapped nerve' is used a lot to describe this sort of
pain.

Radiating pain may be due to bad muscle *spasm*, for
example. This is tightly contracted muscle that is unable
to release, causing pain from:

● lack of circulation
● excess waste fluid build-up and
● pain where tendon knits into bone

Two more words used to describe painful back conditions are *acute* and *chronic*. In everyday language they
are both used to mean 'pretty awful'. Used medically,
though, neither term describes the severity of the problem.

● *Acute* means the pain usually comes on very suddenly
  and is short lived. Official statistics usually state that
  the majority of acute back problems clear up within
  three to five days. If the problem does not resolve fully
  but comes back time and again these bouts of pain are
  known as *recurrent episodes*.
● *Chronic* means the problem usually comes on over a
  period (although its very first appearance may be as
  'acute' back pain) is long-lasting and comes and goes.

Pain and posture

There are pain-sensitive nerve endings sprinkled
throughout the *musculoskeletal system* (the bones, or
skeleton, and muscles which make up the 'frame' of the
body). This is especially true of all the connective tissue
– but the musculoskeletal system is also extremely sensitive to *changes of position*, which are registered by the
nervous system.

There is a constant 'chatter' passing from nerves in
the connective tissue along to the spinal cord. From here,

they pass up to the balance centres of the brain and inner ear. Orders are then sent back to the muscles on the strength of the information received. This results in continuing readjustment of the tension in the muscles that help hold us upright, our postural muscles, and is another way (besides pain) that our bodies have of protecting us against damage.

Sometimes, though, an area of the back can become super-sensitive through high levels of nerve activity, and this is when backs are most prone to everyday injury.

What leads to everyday back injuries?

Just as your brain can ignore pain signals when you are occupied so your mind can dwell on them if you are scared or miserable. In the same way, the brain can choose to ignore or dwell on the signals it receives about the levels of tissue tension in your body.

According to American research during the last decades your brain can literally 'adjust the volume' on selected sections of the spine. This allows it either to ignore the complaints of tight tissues or to become more sensitive to their messages. These adjustments happen during periods of both undue calm and loud complaining in the tension signals reaching the brain.

When the 'nervous chatter' is monitored closely and the volume is turned up the level of reply from the brain is also 'louder'. In other words, the messages running back down to the muscles can cause massive spasm instead of fine balance adjustments.

For example, when your domestic 'Superman' has spent two days successfully moving paving stones and then his back completely seizes on him only when he sits down and reaches forward for a well-deserved cup of tea, he will complain: 'I only went to lift a cup!' But what had really been going on?

Well, for the last two days his 'higher brain' had been

telling his tissue tension monitors to put up with the strains of lifting heavy slabs of stone. The 'volume' had thus had to be turned down. When he sat down at last there was an odd silence on the tension monitors. *Up went the volume.* He leant forward to pick up his cup – and suddenly the 'noise' in the tension monitors would have been deafening. The brain is instantly alarmed and slams the brakes on – in this case the muscles which check his bending forwards. His back is in spasm and he can't move.

He hasn't necessarily damaged anything but he is trapped in a muscular splint, and ignoring this in the same way that he ignored what he was doing to his back earlier may result in damage. (For first aid for acute back pain see Chapter 4.)

The moral is: prepare gradually for heavier jobs and be fit for them in the first place. Don't do jobs which involve repeated bending, twisting and lifting – even the lighter jobs – without taking frequent breaks.

The psychology of pain

So far we have looked at different types of pain. But pain itself is complicated. It is a combination of sensations and responses which include our emotions. Past experiences affect people in different ways. Some get completely 'wound up' at the first hint of a return of a pain they recognize. Others may be flat on their backs unable to move but mentally in control because they understand the cause of their pain. For many people, half the battle is conquering the fears brought on by pain.

The other half of the battle is getting rid of the pain. Let's look at why this is necessary, apart from giving us a feeling of relief.

The negative role of pain

It is well known that pain increases shock. Shock in turn hampers circulation which is so important in healing tissue. Reducing pain will therefore help the healing process.

Pain is also exhausting, and we need extra energy to deal with injury and disease, so pain reduction will increase our energy reserves.

Using natural means of pain relief is very desirable, as the body is already struggling in the face of pain. Hitting it with foreign substances like painkillers is not the only answer (but see box on 'Drugs for back pain' in Chapter 5, p. 65).

The way we cope with pain

People's sensitivity to pain varies greatly. Most people have heard of and use the term 'pain threshold'. This refers to the level of painful input (or *stimuli*) someone needs before they begin to feel pain. A person with a high pain threshold can stand far more painful stimuli before he or she experiences pain, and vice versa. Whether a person has to cope with pain at all, then, depends initially on their pain threshold.

Once the brain or spinal cord pick up pain signals, pain-reducing measures leap into action. What happens is that the brain can send a message to special cells in the spinal cord which dampen these pain stimuli by producing natural painkillers called *endorphins*. There are also special chemicals found in the blood which reduce pain locally.

Research has shown that people with serious wounds, women in labour and athletes can produce high concentrations of endorphins and other natural painkillers. These people seem to feel less pain if they have received positive encouragement from their supporters, be they ambulance staff, midwives or sports trainers. Perhaps this allows them to dip deeper into their instinctive reserves and increase the levels of natural painkillers they produce.

Another natural route to pain relief makes use of the so-called 'gate theory of pain'.

The 'gate theory' of pain

The gate theory, first put forward in 1965, says that pain messages travelling along the nervous system only reach the brain if enough of them reach an imaginary 'gate' and open it. This theory supports the idea that there is a clear pain 'threshold'.

As dull ache-conducting nerve fibres transmit their message relatively slowly, the faster-moving light and firm touch fibres can be activated to beat the pain fibres to the 'gate' and close it behind them. In other words, pleasurable touch is a way of blocking out nagging pain.

Using the gate theory to treat back pain

When we bang ourselves we immediately rub the area to ease the pain, and it works (except for very sharp pains). Other therapies use the same idea to relieve pain, including back pain. They are:

- massage (see Chapter 7)
- acupuncture (see Chapter 9) and
- TENS machines (see Chapter 5)

The causes of back pain

Now that you know more about both backs and pain let's look at your back pain again. You may be one of the 'lucky' ones who know exactly what started it, but even then you may be adding two and two together and making five. There are so many causes of back pain that you cannot easily make your own diagnosis. However, there are symptoms which can point you in the right direction at the right speed, and these are outlined below.

Why you may need to see a doctor

If you are having your first ever attack of back pain you may find it reassuring to see your doctor in any case – if you can get there. Although you may be in a state of shock at how awful it can be, back pain is not normally something you should call your doctor about in the middle of the night. Most acute attacks of back pain subside within three to five days anyway and *nobody can give you an instant cure.*

There are, however, times when you should seek immediate help (see also box on pp. 30–31).

- You may have damaged your spine and need immobilizing, as after a fall or accident.
- There may be severe pressure from, say, a burst disc against your delicate spinal cord (this can cause permanent nerve damage and interfere with the workings of your vital organs if left unattended).
- You may be seriously ill. (Although this is often a fear that accompanies back pain you will normally sense very clearly when you are actually ill.)

There are other times when you should seek medical help, simply because your symptoms point to illness rather than to back problems. You may still get some relief from helping your back but you might be wasting time in not facing the real problem. For example, two causes of back pain that can be fatal if ignored are an *aortic aneurism* (a usually fatal burst of the main artery) and a heart attack.

A heart attack, or *acute myocardial infarction* as doctors call it, normally causes severe chest pain which you cannot pinpoint and which can spread down one arm or up the neck and jaw. This is another example of *referred pain*. A heart attack may come with a feeling of indigestion or back pain.

The pain of a heart attack is impossible to ignore and may also come with any of the following:

- shortness of breath (doctors call this *dyspnoea*, pronounced 'dispnear')

- nausea
- dizziness
- feeling faint
- feeling cold
- feeling very aware of the 'thudding' of your heartbeat
  (or *palpitations*)

Seek urgent medical help if you have these symptoms.

There are times when you might well be so bothered by a pain in your back that you forget about other symptoms which may need medical attention. Make sure you do not fall into this category before you focus on your back.

When to seek immediate medical advice

If, along with pain in your back, you have any of the following symptoms (which point to possible pressure on your spinal cord), get to a doctor quickly.

- Loss of bladder or bowel control; that is, *either*
  - sudden *incontinence* (passing urine or faeces unexpectedly), *or*
  - loss of the normal sensation of wanting to pass urine or have a bowel movement, eventually causing a dangerous 'damming up' of either system.
- Numbness or 'pins and needles' around your *anus* (back passage) or genital organs (taken together these sites are known as the 'saddle area').
- Any weak limbs (not including when pain stops you from putting your foot to the floor). The sort of things you should look out for are *either*
  - a 'giving way' feeling in an arm or leg when you attempt to use it, *or*
  - your foot flops down on to the ground when you take a step, and the foot-lifting muscles don't seem to obey you.
- Muscle-wasting – you may notice one limb seems a lot skinnier than the other (although left and right are never quite the same as the arm and leg we use most will

---

always be a bit thicker) or you may notice one part of a limb seems to have lost its rounded outline and become very 'weedy'.
● Widespread loss of sensation in either or both legs (but not just from sitting awkwardly and cutting off your circulation).

Also consult a doctor for symptoms of ill-health such as:
 – a rash, or other skin changes
 – a high temperature (fever)
 – loss of appetite
 – sudden weight loss for no apparent reason
 – night sweats
 – general weakness
 – drowsiness
 – nausea ('feeling sick')
 – vomiting ('being sick')
 – aversion to bright lights (*photophobia*)
 – severe headache, especially if you have never had one before

Note If you have a *sudden* stiff neck together with *any of the last four symptoms* seek immediate medical help. You could have *meningitis* (inflammation of the coverings of the spinal cord) or a *brain haemorrhage* (a leak of blood inside the skull or brain). These often respond well if caught in time but can be fatal if not.

Non-spinal causes of back pain

There are many problems which can cause back pain other than injury of some kind. Their symptoms, with possible explanations, follow. If you are suffering with any of the symptoms do see your doctor. Although not quite as urgent as the symptoms in the list above, some of these problems can become very nasty if left to develop. You may have one of the following if, as a rule of thumb, your pain is *either*:

- not improved at all, even temporarily, by any change in position, by rest or by movement, *or*
- continuous, troubling you day and night, *or*
- getting steadily worse over a period of weeks or months

Flu or fever

If you have started feeling generally unwell, have a mild fever and widespread aches and pains you may have flu. Flu-like symptoms do often bring back pain with them. This can be caused by the condition itself, as the body uses the joints and muscles as a sort of 'dumping ground' for toxins produced during the fight against disease. These are then cleared away by the lymphatic system (see Chapter 2) once the main fight is won.

The other reason why backache can develop with flu and fever is bed rest. Lying propped up in bed and lack of exercise are both bad news for backs, so do move around gently if you possibly can.

If your temperature is very high, or making you delirious or violently shivery, consult your doctor at once.

Pneumonia and pleurisy

If your back pain comes with pain around your lower ribs (just above waist level) you may be heading for a lung infection. You may feel pain at the tip of one shoulder. If you also begin to develop a cough and a fever and have pain on breathing in, see your doctor as soon as possible.

Ulcers of the stomach and duodenum

Your stomach lies in the upper central part of your abdomen, extending to the left. It is where your food lands after you have chewed it, and where it gets churned up and broken down in a strong acid solution.

The duodenum is a short tube which carries the fluid produced by the stomach into the small intestine.

Both the stomach and duodenum need to maintain a healthy mucus-producing lining to withstand the wear and tear from rough food particles and the strong chemicals which break them down. When this lining is eroded it becomes an *ulcer*. This raw patch of diseased, often bleeding, tissue can cause a burning type of mid-back pain, usually made worse by fatty or spicy foods. (If the ulcer bleeds your bowel movements may look blackish.)

If your back pain varies according to what you eat or drink see your doctor.

Pancreatitis

The pancreas is another digestive organ, and is also vital for keeping a steady sugar balance in the blood. It lies suspended under the stomach, and the enzymes it makes pour into the duodenum along a tiny tube shared with the gallbladder.

If a gallstone blocks this tube, or if you drink too much, your pancreas can become inflamed. This can cause an *intermittent* ('on-and-off') gnawing pain in your mid-back. *This situation can become dangerous if*:

- there is a severe blockage causing back pressure into the pancreas
- an alchoholic 'binge' has resulted in severe inflammation
- a duodenal ulcer has *perforated* (When the ulcer has eroded so that a part of the wall of the duodenum is completely destroyed. This allows the strong pancreatic juices to flow freely around the abdominal organs, wreaking havoc.)

In these cases the back pain will be hard to ignore, and will often come with severe abdominal pain. *This condition needs urgent medical attention.*

Gallbladder problems

The gallbladder hangs just under the liver in the lower right rib-cage, near the front. It produces a fluid called bile, which helps in fat digestion. Because of the ingredients of bile, stones often form here. These may never become a problem but if too many gallstones form, or if the gallbladder becomes inflamed, the gallbladder can become painful. You may feel pain in the lower tip of one shoulder-blade. This may well come with colicky abdominal pains, and possibly fever and shaking.

Consult your doctor if you have any of these symptoms.

Kidney problems

The kidneys sit at the back of the abdomen, just peeking out from below the ribs either side of the spine. Each one is surrounded by a cushion of solid fat to protect it, but they are still very prone to injury from heavy blows to the back.

The job of the kidneys is constantly to filter the body fluids to maintain the fine chemical balance human cells need to survive. The kidneys produce their waste fluid – urine –and retain water from this as required by the body.

Stones can form in the kidneys as they do in the gallbladder and these stones, or any infection, can interfere with these delicate processes. If you have *intermittent* ('off-and-on') colicky and lower back pain along with nausea you may have kidney stones.

If a stone actually blocks a *ureter* (the tube leading from a kidney to the bladder) you will have excruciating abdominal pain, often going into your groin or crotch area.

If your low back pain, with or without abdominal pain, is constant or severe, you have a fever and your urine is discoloured you may well have a kidney infection. Drink plenty of good clean *water* and see your doctor soon.

Gynaecological problems

Because of the nerve supply from the lower back to the female reproductive organs – that is, ovaries, uterus (or womb), fallopian tubes (which carry eggs from the ovary to the womb), cervix (the neck of the womb) and vagina (the birth canal) – women can suffer particular problems of back pain. Any gynaecological disorder can refer pain to that area of the back.

Period pain (which doctors also call *menstrual pain*), uterine cramps and premenstrual tension can cause a *diffuse* (spread-out) low back pain severe enough to interfere with all normal activities. Do what feels best at these times. Normally rest, gentle exercise or a hot water bottle will help.

Pregnancy often brings bouts of back pain with it. One of the reasons is that the pregnancy hormones make all the connective tissues much more elastic, starting very early on in the pregnancy. This makes it possible for a woman's body to be wonderfully stretchy for the birth, but it also makes her prone to overstretching before the event. The joints of the pelvis are especially at risk.

A *prolapsed womb*, when the ligaments in the uterus stretch and allow the womb to drop down into the vagina, can produce a dull, dragging low backache, besides putting pressure on the bladder.

An infection of the womb or fallopian tubes (the general term for these infections is *pelvic inflammatory disease*, or PID) can also cause back pain. This may come with abdominal pain, vaginal discharge or pain during lovemaking.

Most of these sources of backache have other clear symptoms as well so are hard to confuse with back injury. If your symptoms are severe, consult your doctor.

Spinal injuries needing medical attention

By now you should be reasonably clear whether you are
unwell or not, and whether you need to see your doctor
before looking either at self-help or treatment for your
back pain. But there are still a few situations we need to
look at with caution. These are serious and unstable back
injuries and they can be dangerous if left untreated.

Spinal cord damage
If you have been in a car accident or had a fall or jolt in
the last day or two and are getting:

- any of the first batch of symptoms in the box 'When to
  seek immediate medical advice', pp. 30–31
- weakness in any limbs, or
- difficulty in controlling your limb muscles since the
  injury

you may have some damage to your spinal cord. *This
needs to be looked at urgently.*

Damage to the ribs
If you have been hit in your back or rib-cage, whether
from a fight, fooling about or falling, beware of pain on
breathing in. You may have:

- a cracked or broken rib (very little can be done about
  this particular situation, but at least if you know that
  you have damaged ribs you can be very careful about
  how you move to prevent any sharp ends puncturing
  your lung)
- more serious spinal injury

Crush fracture of a vertebra
If you have had a violent injury, or have had no external
injury but are elderly and develop a sudden severe disabling pain (usually in the mid-back or lower back), a
vertebra may have collapsed entirely. An x-ray will
show a wedge-shaped vertebra causing a visible kink in

the painful area. You may be bent forwards, with pain radiating round to both sides of your chest or abdomen. Again, medical attention is obviously needed.

Coccydinia
If you have fallen on to your tailbone (or *coccyx*, pronounced 'cocksix'), and have:

- a persistent sensation of bruising
- difficulty sitting comfortably
- pain in the coccyx area during bowel motions

you may have *coccydinia*. This normally heals given time but if the pain is intense a doctor may prescribe a pain-relieving injection or suppository (a special form of pain-reliever inserted into the anus) as immediate first aid (but see also homoeopathic first aid remedies in Chapter 4, pp. 50–51). If the pain does not disappear over a few months you may need manipulation from an *osteopath* or *chiropractor* (see Chapter 7). Only very occasionally does the condition require surgery.

Less serious spinal conditions

The following spinal conditions may need medical attention or the attentions of a specialist natural therapist.

Damage to the discs
Acute disc prolapse This is when the outer wall of the intervertebral disc ruptures allowing the inner gel to press on surrounding tissues. Disc problems occur most often in the lower back, occasionally in the neck, and rarely in the thoracic spine (usually, because the ribs serve as stabilizers, only as a result of violent injury). Symptoms vary enormously depending on where the protrusion is pressing but those which can point to disc damage are pain down one or both legs which is made worse by coughing, sneezing or laughing.

Treatment by careful manipulation, massage and traction can hasten recovery and prevent long-term patterns of muscle tension from becoming 'locked in' to your back. Very occasionally surgery is necessary – for example, to remove floating pieces of disc which have not been reabsorbed from the spinal canal.

Chronic disc prolapse Sometimes discs are in a bad state and keep bulging out of line, usually aggravated by bending, lifting and twisting. Aching and stiffness after compressing the spine (as in sitting) are often part of this usually middle-aged symptom picture.

Again, gentle manipulation, massage, acupuncture and re-education of your posture will help. This problem improves in old age as the discs dry out and the ligaments harden.

General tissue damage

Scar tissue Although it serves an essential purpose, scar tissue in the wrong place or in the wrong amounts can be a real menace to backs. It is a strong, rather inelastic mending material. (You can see it wherever your skin has been badly damaged.) It forms as part of the 'knitting-up' process of any broken, cut, torn or badly inflamed tissue, be it skin, muscle, bone, nerve or connective tissue. At first, the body normally makes too much of it, and then reabsorbs it very slowly. Fresh scar tissue is sticky and can cause *adhesions*, gluing the wrong layers together and stopping them from gliding smoothly against each other. Old scar tissue, by contrast, is often hard and tender, causing local fluid stagnation and widespread long-term changes in body tensions.

Many back problems are thought to be caused by areas of repeated straining and scarring. Where this happens outside the spinal canal – that is, in the back muscles and reasonably accessible ligaments – the manual therapies can help a great deal to break it down, particularly skilled massage using deep friction.

Whiplash syndrome Any accident, for example in a car, in which you are unexpectedly shunted forward from behind is called a 'whiplash'. This is because your spine is briefly forced to flick forwards, and reacts by snapping backwards just like a cracking whip. Your head is on the end of this whip, and so most of the strain is taken by the soft tissues of your neck. But it can affect your whole spine, right down to the sacrum.

Early treatment of symptoms coming on after a jolt like this is recommended.

Damage to nerves

Nerve compression This normally means pressure on the spinal nerve roots within the spinal canal or intervertebral foramina from any source – bone, ligament or nerve sheath scarring, disc wall or nucleus. It can also mean pressure on any spinal nerve along its course through the back: it could be held by a spasm in the buttock, for example, which is a very common source of *sciatica*. Nerve compression can also happen as a result of a nerve being 'tethered' (or 'glued') by scar tissue if it heals badly. Symptoms vary according to location but can track from the spine down one arm or leg. You may also feel tingling or numbness.

If the cause of the compression lies outside the spinal canal, manual therapy can usually help (see Chapter 7), but if the cause of the problem lies within the spinal canal this condition can be hard to clear up, and may mean quite a lot of adjustment in your activities. Any therapy which improves the circulation may help to alleviate inflammation. Gentle exercise, specific stretching and avoiding painful activities and positions may also help. You may be advised to have steroid injections to give short-term relief. Surgery is a last resort as it can itself cause scarring (see Chapter 5, p. 78).

Nerve root fibrosis If a spinal nerve has suffered inflammation or bruising from a disc or bony protrusion, its connective tissue sleeve may become scarred (or *fibrosed*). This may make it too bulky for its own space, or it may have become stuck to the walls of the spinal canal. Pain will normally occur when the scarred portion is compressed, or the stuck part is stretched.

Getting out of the position which brought on the pain normally helps. Again, a long-term programme of improving spinal circulation and mobility may help.

Joint strains

These are common in the spine – because there are so many joints in the first place and because of the way we misuse our backs. Pain is usually around the affected joint, and may be aggravated by weight-bearing and the particular movements which stress the damaged tissues.

The following are examples of joint strains commonly treated very successfully by natural therapists:

- *Facet joint strain* This can feel like a 'bone out of place'.
- *Rib joint strain* This often comes with pain radiating round your chest from the back.
- *Sacroiliac joint strain* This is pain around the 'dimple' area of one buttock, which may feel like or 'mimic' *sciatica*.
- *Slack or chronically strained ligaments* Where joints have been strained repeatedly or overstretched (as in high-level gymnastics and ballet) the ligaments stop limiting them effectively. Treatment needs to be aimed at improving stability. This is much trickier to sort out than freeing an area that is stuck so prevention is clearly the best medicine here.

Problems with bones

These cover anything from the tiniest crack in a bone to a major 'slippage' of a damaged vertebra. Orthopaedic specialists (doctors who specialize in the treatment of bones) are there to help with serious damage but minute fractures are hard to pick up on x-ray and mostly just need time to heal.

Problems with muscles

Actual muscle damage to your back is not as common as you might expect. It usually occurs suddenly during or after vigorous sport as a result of not warming up or cooling down properly. Muscular problems which are common and will usually respond well to the natural approach are:

- uneven muscle tension from habit, misuse, or badly repaired injury
- hardening (*fibrosis*) from prolonged lack of use for whatever reason
- congestion (lack of local circulation) from chronic tightness

Deformities

Minor deformities of the spine are quite common and may never cause any symptoms. If you have one like a marked sideways curve (called a *scoliosis*) which you feel is setting up a tension pattern through your back, a regular visit to an osteopath or chiropractor may be very useful.

Mild to moderate childhood deformities may be helped dramatically by regular visits to a *cranial osteopath* who gently helps to guide the growing tissues to reach their full potential.

If you have serious deformities, these will have been spotted by the time you read this book, and treated by orthopaedic specialists and physiotherapists. Natural therapies can also often be a great help by keeping you soft and supple in different ways.

Problems of ageing

In time our spines do 'tell our story' – some more loudly than others. The following are terms which label common conditions of so-called *degeneration*. This may sound like a slippery slope but it happens to all of us and does not necessarily cause pain.

- *Spondylosis* This means arthritic changes in the vertebrae and their joints.
- *Spondylitis* This is inflammation of one or more vertebrae.
- *Osteophytes* These are little 'cliff edges' on the vertebral bodies. These may jut into the nerve spaces at the sides leading to a feeling of the nerve being 'pinched', maybe with tingling or numbness. This is usually helped by sitting or being bent forwards, which gives the nerves more space. Sometimes these bony spurs jut back centrally into the spinal canal and press on the spinal cord, usually in the lower back. (For symptoms of spinal cord compression see box above on 'When to seek immediate medical advice', pp. 30–31).
- *Osteoporosis* This is thinning of the bones from disuse after illness or injury, from bad diet or, in women, hormonal changes after the menopause. Symptoms only appear if the bones begin to break easily, normally very late in life (see 'Crush fracture of a vertebra' above). Specific bone-loading exercises and a 'good back diet' (see chapter 4, pp. 55–60) are the best prevention.

Inflammatory diseases that affect the spine

These are common diseases that involve the whole body and cause back pain in special ways.

- *Rheumatoid arthritis* This leads eventually to weakened ligaments throughout the body and makes any vigorous manipulation unsafe, but gentle mobilizing to help lymphatic drainage and keep joints mobile is a good idea.

● *Ankylosing spondylitis* This is an inflammatory condition mostly affecting young men. It centres around the spine and its neighbouring joints in the ribs and pelvis. The symptoms, x-rays and blood tests confirm the diagnosis. It has phases of acute inflammation followed by a gradual stiffening of the whole spine (called *calcification*). Again, manipulation of hardened spines is not a good idea but plenty of exercise and gentle mobilizing is essential.

(See also *The Natural Way With Arthritis and Rheumatism*.)

Summary

Back pain can have many different symptoms and causes, some of them serious. Common sense is the best guide to understanding and diagnosing your particular back pain. Most back pain caused by disease will give you other pains and make you feel rotten into the bargain.

Doctors are always on the lookout for signs of disease – but so are well-trained natural therapists. They have to study diseases just as doctors do in case you need the attentions of a specialist. So you need have no fear in seeing one so long as they are fully and properly qualified (see Chapter 10).

It is still true, though, that the vast majority of back pain is caused by some kind of build-up of tension or trauma to the tissues. These problems can so often be better helped without heavyweight medical intervention but rather with the help of the many gentle natural treatments, some of which you can do for yourself. We'll look at those next.

CHAPTER 4

How to help yourself

Tips and guidelines for prevention and treatment

Taking positive steps to maintain your health is a very important part of natural medicine. It is called prevention and is the main subject of this chapter.

Preventive measures don't always stop our backs from hurting at some point in our lives, though. These painful phases happen because we have overstrained our backs without realizing it, or because we have been neglecting ourselves during a crisis that has demanded our full attention. Tension builds up unnoticed and our backs take the strain.

When this happens you probably want to see someone right away in the hope that they can help you. But there are actually quite a few things you can do for yourself that might take the problem away entirely – *and* the need to spend money on treatment. So here are some useful self-help tips for you to try before seeking professional help, not only to keep back pain at bay but also to help an existing problem.

If you are in pain right now

You may not be in the mood to read much because your back is simply too painful to concentrate. Even if you read nothing else, though, you should check through the box on 'When to seek immediate medical advice' in Chapter 3, p. 30, because it shows you how to recognize symptoms of back pain that may need urgent or expert attention.

First aid for sore backs

Now that you have reassured yourself that you are not in any immediate danger let's look at what simple 'first aid' steps you can take right away to ease the problem and any pain. The choice between the following options may seem straightforward but each has its good and its bad points. No two backs are the same so you may need to try a combination of them – either at the same time or one after the other – before you hit on a solution that is right for you.

Bed rest

This used to be the instant answer to back pain in many cases but not any more. There are good and bad points about resting up for back pain and you can make up your own mind by using the following lists to come to a sensible decision:

Good points about bed rest

● It takes the combined pressure of gravity and your body weight off your spine and this can relieve pain if it is caused by a bulging disc. (The effect of standing upright is to *double* the pressure on your discs.)
● It relaxes the postural muscles of the neck, back and pelvis, which again can reduce muscle tension and relieve pressure on spinal nerves.
● It lessens the irritation of inflamed tissues. If a nerve is surrounded by toxic chemicals around a damaged area which is healing, or nipped by the pressure of a bony spur which has developed next to it, the nerve becomes swollen and inflamed. The last thing it needs is to be tweaked and twisted with hefty weights on top of it. It needs time to heal. Just as you would rest a sprained wrist until it feels more comfortable once the swelling goes down, a sprained spinal joint needs rest too.

After looking at these three points, you might feel like flopping into bed and letting nature do the rest. Nature gets up to some sneaky tricks, though, while your injured back is lying still.

Bad points about bed rest

● It leads to rapid muscle-wasting which weakens the back. This, in turn, makes the back even more prone to injury.

● It hampers the circulation which relies on active movement to boost the activity of the heart (see Chapter 2 'The importance of exercise'). This in turn slows down the healing and drainage of damaged, swollen and congested tissues.

● It promotes the formation of scar tissue. Injured tissues literally do their own darning: whenever there is tissue damage blood rushes to the area (hence the swelling) and forms a clot. Within 24 hours a sticky mesh of protein called *fibrin* combines with cells which weave new fibrous tissue within this clot. If damaged muscles or ligaments are moved about as they heal the fibrous tissue is laid down in the correct order along the lines of force created by these movements. But if the damaged tissues are kept slack (by lying in bed) the fibrous scar tissue is deposited in a haphazard way, sticking layers together right, left and centre. Muscles get stuck together, bones get stuck to ligaments, and these 'adhesions' become a painful nuisance in years to come.

So, in general, if you do feel you need bed rest the lesson is to keep yourself moving 'a little and often', as often as half-hourly if you possibly can, but within sensible limits. That means don't overdo it. Let the pain tell you when to stop. Too much pain is overdoing it.

Traction

This means stretching the spine along its length to ease muscle spasm and take pressure off the discs. There are two sorts of traction, horizontal and vertical.

Horizontal traction

This is hard to achieve at home as you need to apply a pulling force at either or both ends of you (see Chapter 5, p. 71). You can do it, though, in the following ways.

- For an aching neck try stretching it yourself. Lie down and let your head rest on your cupped hands. Tuck the sides of your thumbs under the base of your skull and gently stretch out the upper neck muscles. Now concentrate on relaxing your neck and letting it lengthen. You may find, as you relax, that you need to slide your hands a little further up the bed to increase the stretch and 'take up the slack'.
- For low back pain you will need a friend to help you: lie flat while your helper holds under your ankles and lifts your legs up to a comfortable angle and stretches them gently. Your helper may find this easier by gripping your ankles firmly and leaning back slowly. In this position lazy, rhythmic swinging of your legs from side to side will help undo lower back tightness.
- In the absence of a willing helper lie on your back with your legs draped, knees bent, over a fulcrum like a beach ball or a pile of pillows. This will again stretch your lower back. Concentrate on allowing your back to lengthen. Tucking a rolled-up towel into your waist can help a lot, too, even in a semi-sitting position.

Vertical traction

You can apply this to your back in an upright position or upside-down like a bat. For upside-down traction you will need 'anti-gravity' ankle boots or a device called a 'Backswing'.

For thoracic or lower back pain, provided your shoulders feel all right, try hanging upright by your arms from a door, an overhead beam or horizontal bar. Drape a towel over the top of a wide-open door (or beam etc) as near the hinges as possible (so you don't rip the door off). Rest your front against the door and reach up in front of you gripping the top of the door firmly with both hands through the towel. Slowly bend your knees, keeping your feet on the ground and your spine as relaxed as possible, and hold that position. Your arms will tire quite quickly so rest and repeat several times.

For chronic pain from the effects of compression anywhere along your spine (spinal degeneration, tension, gravity, lifting and so on) consider a backswing. This is a tilting frame (also known as *inversion therapy*) on which you hang, again by your ankles, but which allows you to adjust the angle of tilt from horizontal to vertical. Many users have reported great relief from using this topsy-turvy contraption, but beware: *never hang upside-down if you suffer from high blood pressure, heart disease, recent strokes, 'drop attacks', glaucoma, conjunctivitis or retinal detachment* – in other words from heart, blood vessel or eye problems.

Mechanical support

This often seems like a mixed blessing, even when you are in pain. But spinal corsets, support belts and cervical (neck) collars do have two distinct advantages.

- They stop some of the bending, twisting and jarring movements that may be damaging to your healing back.
- Corsets and support belts increase the pressure within your abdomen which gives support to your spine (much like holding your breath before lifting a heavy weight).

A much simpler method of providing a reminder not to bend and twist, though, is to get someone to stick a few long strips of non-stretch sticking plaster from shoulder blade to buttock level or across your lower back and pelvis, or both! (Pharmacies sell special fluids these days which make taking off plasters painless if that's a worry.)

Supports, especially heavy spinal corsets, have most of the disadvantages of bed rest with none of its advantages – that is, reduced pressure on the discs and protection of the spinal nerves from irritating tugs. Supports should *not* be used *except* in the first few days of a back injury and for no more than six weeks unless under the guidance of a specialist.

Pain relief

Conventional pain relief is discussed at length in Chapter 5. This includes the names of over-the-counter drugs, their effects and side-effects. In general it is fine to use these for a few days but you should seek advice from your doctor or a natural therapist specializing in back pain if your symptoms persist. The same goes for the following natural remedies.

● *Fish oil* This includes salmon, halibut and cod liver oil. Unlike many diets and vitamins fish oil has been scientifically compared with drug therapy for the relief of inflammation. One recent Swedish study concluded that 10g (0.35oz) of fish oil a day had similar anti-inflammatory powers to conventional drugs (NSAIDs – see Chapter 5). Another study in Scotland showed that rheumatoid arthritis sufferers (whose main problem is pain from inflammation) could reduce their NSAID dosages without any worsening of their symptoms by taking fish oils. Fish oils are widely available in chemists and health food stores. *But a word of warning:* excessive fish oils in quantities can lead to changes in white blood cell counts and *may* cause bleeding in the brain.

- *Herbs* Herbs said to be effective for pain relief in general include *guaiacum, Jamaican dogwood, St John's wort* and *valerian.* 'Anti-inflammatories', which claim to treat the underlying causes of back pain, include *black willow, devil's claw, meadowsweet, white poplar* and *wild yam.* But such a vast selection of herbs is claimed to be effective, and their exact application in conditions involving the back is so complex, that a visit to an experienced and qualified medical herbalist is really essential.

Homoeopathy

This offers some of the safest, most gentle (and cheapest) remedies for back pain.

Homoeopathic remedies for back pain

To find a homoeopathic self-help remedy for back pain choose, from the following list, the one that describes your symptoms most closely.

Arnica montana:
- for any problem arising from an injury like a fall, an accident, whiplash or concussion
- for any back pain with bruising and soreness – even the ill-effects of old injuries can be helped by arnica

Rhus toxicodendron (or *Rhus tox* for short):
- for pain and stiffness extending into the big muscles of the back, typically worse after resting and when first starting to move, and better from continuing to move
- backs that seize up after lifting or moving heavy objects

Ruta graveolens (*Ruta grav*):
- for pain focussed along the spine itself (similar to *Rhus tox;* a good choice if the pains are worse for rest and better for getting moving)

Hypericum:
- for nagging pains in the tail-end of the spine, for example after a fall or after a difficult birth

Bellis perennis:
- for low back pain in the later months of pregnancy (first be sure you are not in labour, though)

Symphytum:
- for fractures, to help them heal better and more quickly

Homoeopathic remedies come in small white tablets in a variety of strengths or *potencies*. In the UK the most common potency is labelled '6' or '6c'. The tablets need to dissolve in your mouth rather than be swallowed. Take one tablet three times a day until the pain improves, when the dosage should be reduced or stopped. (The labels on tubs of homoeopathic remedies often suggest taking two tablets at a time. While this does make the tablets – and your money – disappear more quickly it does not have the same effect on your pain!). All the above remedies can be bought at most good pharmacies and health food shops, or can be ordered from a homoeopathic pharmacy or specialist supplier. For more on homoeopathy see Chapter 9, p. 119.

Hydrotherapy

Hydrotherapy is treatment using water and is one of the very oldest forms of therapy known.

Ice packs

These help to reduce pain from swelling and inflammation from a *recent* injury (one that happened less than 48 hours ago). They are less useful if the injury is old. Either use a pack of frozen peas or sweetcorn wrapped in a wet tea towel or buy a special gel-pack for the purpose from a pharmacy or sports shop. (Unlike peas, gel-packs can also be warmed up and used as a hot pack.) Apply the pack to the injury for no more than 20 minutes. If you need to repeat the process wait for 20 minutes before re-applying the pack (but don't forget to put the frozen food back in the deep-freeze meanwhile: alternatively you can use two packs alternately). Do this for no longer than two hours and then wait two hours before starting again.

Hot packs
These help to increase circulation into areas of stiffness and injury by widening blood vessels. A number of normal household items can be used very effectively for this, such as:

- a covered hot-water bottle
- a gel-pack
- a heat pad or lamp
- a sock full of rock salt warmed in the oven

Apply the pack to the painful area as needed and try to stretch gently afterwards.

Hot and cold contrast bathing
This a method of using first hot water and then cold to stimulate the circulation of blood around an injury *after* the first 48 hours. It has been a traditional treatment for sports injuries for as long as anyone can remember. Hold the affected part under a shower of water for a minute as hot as you can stand and then splash with cold water for another half a minute. Continue this bracing process for five to ten minutes. People who do this recover better than those who don't.

Steam
The easiest way to apply steam to your back is by using a towel. Soak a hand towel in the hottest water you can bear and wring it out (if you can). If your back is too painful for this ask for help: it is worth the effort. Place the towel over the painful area and cover the steaming towel with a dry one. This is one of the best methods for 'wry neck' (or *torticollis*) when your neck seizes up com-

pletely. You can increase the effects by spreading a good layer of arnica cream over the painful area first.

Hot baths with essential oils
Hot baths with *essential oils*, the concentrated oils used in *aromatherapy* (see Chapter 7), are a wonderful way to ease general muscle tension and ache. Oils traditionally used for this purpose include rosemary, wintergreen, eucalyptus, camphor and lavender. They are readily available these days from most good health and beauty shops, pharmacists and healthfood shops. Add a few drops to running bath water. There are a number of preparations on the market that use mineral salts (including a natural version from the Dead Sea) to achieve much the same results.

Rubs and sprays

Any number of commercially available products are on the market for quick relief from back pain, from freezing gels and sprays to warming embrocations. They are all highly effective at giving short-term relief quite safely, if expensively, by basically the same principles as the hydrotherapy methods outlined above – that is, by stimulating a rapid flow of blood to the affected part.

What to do after first aid

So much for the first aid. If the suggestions above have helped, you will by now be feeling much better. Your main interest now is to stay pain free and, hopefully, to prevent the pain ever arising again. Although no one can guarantee this, the following tips and guidelines should help you go a long way towards it.

Don't be put off by talk of people who say that if you are past middle age, you are too old for prevention. While it is true that the older you are the more wear and tear will have taken place in your spine, research shows that an enormous number of people in exactly the same situation can lead active lives without so much as a hint of back pain by following such advice.

Even if an x-ray, for example, has shown your spine to be worn (doctors call it 'degenerated') and possibly even labelled 'arthritic' as a result, remember you were pain free for a long time when your spine was just as worn and so there is absolutely no reason to believe you could not be again. Don't give in to a label!

The following measures are long-term ones you can take to improve the state of your back for the rest of your life. They take time and patience and you may be surprised at how much effort you need to make at first. You may need to look at more books, listen to tapes, get in some basic equipment or go to regular classes. But the end result will all be worth it because you will not only be saving yourself a deal of misery but are likely to extend your active life considerably.

The first thing of all is to decide you are going, from this minute on, to be kind to your back. Tell it so. Say from now on you will be sensible and considerate and not take it for granted but give it all the support it needs to keep you fit and healthy.

The next step is to decide to start to be positive about your back by doing two most important things: exercising and relaxing.

Exercising

Exercising for backs has the following aims:

- to help you lose excess weight
- to strengthen your abdominal muscles (these connect your rib-cage to your pelvis at the front and sides and help share any weight your back is carrying)
- to stretch your back, neck and shoulders to reduce tension

Losing weight

Too much weight puts an unnecessary strain on your back from the sheer force of gravity. Statistics show clearly that seriously overweight people have more problems with their weight-bearing joints – knees, hips and spines in particular – than other people. So it obviously makes sense to lose those surplus pounds (it's good for you in other ways too: your heart for example). Losing weight means burning up more than you feed in until you reach a comfortable weight – and then sticking with those new habits for the rest of your life. Reverting to old habits simply means you'll put the pounds straight back on.

Common causes of overweight are:

- sitting around too much doing nothing (watching TV, for example)
- eating too much (of anything but especially too much of the wrong foods such as processed, sweet and fatty foods)
- eating for reasons other than giving yourself energy (for example, 'comfort eating')
- drinking too much (alcoholic drinks like beer contain lots of calories)

So obviously the way to lose weight is to do something about all the above. As far as eating and drinking goes, just cutting down, sensibly, is enough for many people. But the following is the more strenuous approach if you decide you need it:

- First, run out of excuses for *not* losing weight.
- Picture yourself as you would like to be (but be realistic: not everybody can have a model figure nor should they think they need to).
- Start cutting down gradually but relentlessly on all fats, sugars and processed foods in your diet (this

means goodbye to pastries, cakes, biscuits and pre-packed meals).
- Do the same with your intake of alcohol and all fizzy soft drinks (like colas).
- Cut down also on the amount of red meat you eat and avoid, particularly, all animal fat (so don't eat any visible fat in beef, bacon, pork and so on, or the outer skin of poultry like chicken or duck).
- Grill, steam or bake food rather than fry it.
- Eat plenty of fresh fruit and vegetables, particularly green vegetables. (Sprouting seeds such as alfalfa and dry seeds like sunflower, sesame and pumpkin are also all extremely high in the nutrients the body needs for maximum health.)
- Drink plenty of good clean water and fruit and vegetable juice (our body needs about 4 pints/2 litres a day to keep healthy). It is a good idea to dilute fruit juices you buy in the supermarket – even unsweetened ones are high in fruit sugar.
- Exercise.

Exercise is vital to the process of losing weight because dietary changes alone don't usually achieve lasting results.

Ideally we should all exercise 20–30 minutes *at least* three times a week. This means working yourself hard enough to get hot and be out of breath. Known as *aerobic exercising*, this can consist of jogging, cycling, swimming, playing tennis, *hard* walking, mini-trampolining or whatever takes your fancy and sounds fun. Joining an exercise class is fun for some people while swimming is an excellent exercise for those with mobility problems.

However, make sure you are fit for your sport and don't go from the extreme of being a couch potato one minute to throwing yourself into a game of squash the

next. *You could put a fatal strain on your heart this way.*
Work into exercise gently but steadily. If in doubt consult your family doctor or a good fitness instructor (most gyms and health and fitness centres have one) and ask for a health check first.

The secrets of successful dieting

A quick way to lose weight is to stop eating. The problem with 'crash dieting', as it is called, is that it gives completely the wrong signals to your body based on instincts programmed into us aeons ago. It effectively tells your body to prepare for a famine. So when you take up eating again after the diet your body starts laying down fat stores – sometimes making you fatter, and heavier, than you were in the first place.

Another problem is that dieting can also cause too drastic a reduction in your essential mineral intake. This can result in minerals such as calcium and magnesium being leached out of your bones – leading eventually to serious weakening of bones. Bone weakness is called *osteoporosis* and is particularly prevalent in older women, resulting in the characteristic bent back of many old people. More seriously, it also leads to increased likelihood of bones breaking.

The secret of successful dieting is actually a combination of sensible – that means *nutritious* – eating and drinking *and exercise*. Exercise is vital to make sure weight you take off stays off.

The most important vitamins and minerals for a healthy back are folic acid, vitamin C, vitamin D, calcium, magnesium and manganese. Eating plenty of *fresh* fruit and vegetables – particularly green leafy and purple-coloured vegetable (such as beetroot and red cabbage) – will give you most of what you need but it's probably worth boosting your levels temporarily with some good quality food supplements if you have a back problem. Appendix B has recommended reading on both nutritious eating and exercise.

Abdominal muscles

Having good abdominal muscle tone is important whether our lifestyles are strenuous or not. Tone is frequently lost in women after childbirth or in people who sit a lot, have been stuck in bed for a time through illness or injury, spend long hours driving, or are too fat. You can strengthen these important 'back stabilizers' safely and effectively by doing the following (*see figure 5*):

- think about them as often as you can whether standing in a queue, sitting in a car or shopping and just pull them in a little at regular intervals
- do 'the pelvic tilt' when you get up and before you get into bed
- do 'crunches' the same way, a few each morning and night.

If you have difficulty strengthening your abdominal muscles in spite of these exercises try seeing a therapist called an *applied kinesiologist* (see Chapter 7). Your abdominals may be 'switched off' and a kinesiologist, who specializes in testing muscle strengths, may be able to 'reactivate' them.

Stretching

Stretching your back, neck and shoulders to relieve or release tension in the muscles and ligaments does *not* mean putting your body into some painful position and then moving even further into yet more pain! To see true stretching watch a cat: see how it lengthens itself *slowly* to a comfortable maximum and often stays there for a while.

A cat's method of stretching bears out the very latest research. This has shown the little fibres that give connective tissue their elasticity or 'stretchiness' (called the *collagen* fibres) behave in a special way. Before they are stretched they lie dispersed throughout body tissues all higgledy-piggledy, but if they are stretched – so that the

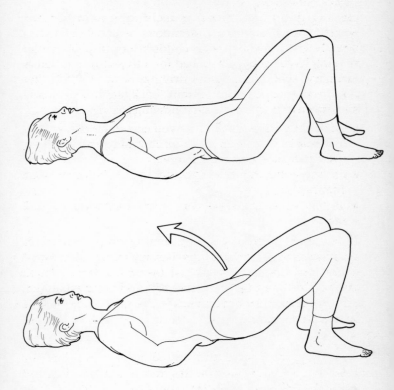

The pelvic tilt

Lie on your back on a comfortable surface somewhere, knees bent, and place one hand under the small of your back, palm down. Keeping your backside on the floor tilt your hips towards your nose. This should squash your hand in the small of your back against the floor. Hold for a few seconds, breathing gently, then slowly release. Repeat this several times.

Fig 5. Abdominal exercises

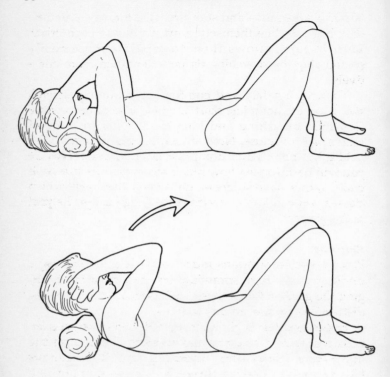

Crunching

Lie down as for the tilt exercise, knees bent, and put a small
support such as a rolled-up towel under your neck. Breathe in,
but don't hold your breath. Cup your hands over your ears,
elbows together, and raise your upper body *a few inches* off
the floor, breathing all the time. As you breathe in again relax
gently and let your neck lie back on to your neck support. You
can vary this exercise by moving towards one knee, then to the
centre, then to the other knee, relaxing back down between
each 'crunch'.

Fig 5. Abdominal exercises

'slack' is taken up – and stay stretched for, say, a minute they begin to line themselves up parallel to each other. This, in turn, allows them to separate more easily so allowing the stretching tissue to lengthen more effectively.

To stretch safely and comfortably yourself, stretch *slowly* up to a point just *short* of when it becomes painful. Continue breathing and hold the stretch for a good while, say a minute. Now stretch a little further. Don't hold it but relax. After doing this a few times every day you will be surprised how much more you can stretch. If you'd rather have someone guide you there are stretch classes you can join at health clubs. Yoga is also helpful in this respect.

Relaxing

Proper relaxation means much more than just having a drink, seeing a film, sprawling on the sofa or even digging the garden. Often these are little more than passing distractions from everyday worries.

Real relaxation is giving your body and mind a complete rest from the strains and tensions that accumulate in everyone from living – including from the chemicals like *adrenalin* flooding through us from our normal, instinctive 'fight or flight' responses to pressures of all sorts, from the boss and bank manager to children and partners.

The overall effect of all this on your muscles, and particularly your back muscles, is to make them tighten up. Little by little prolonged tension of this sort creates a kind of body 'armour' that can hold you in a silent vice, making you both uncomfortable and prone to injury. The secret of relaxing is finding effective ways of shedding this armour.

Both diet and exercise can help – for example both tea and coffee contain chemicals (*caffeine* and *theine*) that work a bit like adrenalin on the body and can aggravate tension – but the most effective methods involve techniques that combine gentle physical movement with mental tranquillity.

For example, meditation and yoga are both excellent ways of teaching yourself to relax properly. Both can be done with the help of the many books and tapes on the market though many people prefer to join a class. Alexander Technique is another method that can help. All involve learning special techniques of breathing, balancing, stretching, calming down, thinking and 'being' that will help you reach quite profound levels of relaxation if you let them. For more details on these methods see Chapters 7–9.

Summary

Sufferers from back pain are often surprised just how much it is within their power to help themselves not only to relieve pain but to remove it altogether – and this realization is often the only tool they need, together with the suggestions in this chapter, for controlling their problem completely.

But sometimes this isn't enough and the help and support of an experienced and sympathetic healthcare professional of one sort or another is the slightly stronger tool needed to achieve the desired result. If you fall into this group, the following chapters will help.

CHAPTER 5

Conventional treatments and approaches

What your doctor is likely to say and do

Conventional methods of helping back pain usually start with a visit to your doctor. If you have had an accident you may find yourself being examined by a hospital doctor. Either way their method of making a diagnosis (that is, deciding what is wrong with you) will be broadly similar. It will consist of:

- taking a case history
- giving you a physical examination

Taking a case history
Doctors will want to know quite a lot of information about you and your pain before deciding what to do next. They will ask you all about your past medical history and write these details down. If you are in a lot of pain this might make you impatient but bear with them. The case history is the first important stage in weeding out serious problems.

The physical examination
After taking the case history the doctor will want to examine you. This means first taking a good look at you so you will need to undress to your underwear (your

back extends from your head to your toes, don't forget!). He will check the movements of your joints and feel for any tender areas. He may also examine your nervous system by tapping some tendons and testing your skin sensitivity.

After the examination your doctor should discuss his findings with you. He will then either offer you direct help or send you for more tests elsewhere.

Direct help your doctor might offer you

Your doctor has various options and may offer you one or more of the following:

- advice on bed rest, or rest on a firm surface
- advice on work – for example, taking time off, returning to lighter duties or even changing jobs
- advice on how to cope better with personal problems such as, for example, debts if financial stress is part of your problem. (One far-sighted British family practice has just hired someone who knows their way around the state benefit system in order to sort out patients' money troubles. As a result the doctors found a great reduction in symptoms – including back pain – which at first were thought to be medical problems!)
- a sheet of 'do's and don'ts' for backs
- referral to a specialist such as an orthopaedic consultant, a rheumatologist or a neurologist (see below for more on specialists)
- referral to a suitable physical therapist – most likely a physiotherapist, or possibly an osteopath, a chiropractor or a massage therapist
- manipulation (more and more doctors are now training in these skills)
- pain relief in the form of medication (see box on 'Drugs for back pain')

Drugs for back pain

There is a wide range of drugs for pain. The most commonly-used are as follows:

Analgesics ('painkillers')

Aspirin*
- is both painkiller and *anti-inflammatory* (helps reduce inflammation)
- is known to cause gut irritation and bleeding, so take with food. Some brands now buffer aspirin with a form of antacid, but this contains aluminium.
- is forbidden to children under the age of 12 except in special cases

Paracetamol*
- is a painkiller but not an anti-inflammatory
- is better for sensitive stomachs
- is passed as safe for use in pregnancy
- is highly poisonous (in large doses it causes liver failure)

Codeine*
Usually sold in combination with aspirin or paracetamol in the same pill, although there is no known benefit to these *compound preparations*.
- useful for mild to moderate pain relief
- comes from opium, and can therefore slow down all normal muscular processes
- too constipating for long-term use
- causes drowsiness
- addictive

Dihydro-codeine tartrate
This is a stronger painkiller, for the relief of moderate to severe pain.

Meptazinol (UK brand name 'Meptid') and
buprenorphine ('Temgesic')
These are also made from the opium poppy and are used to treat severe pain.

Other drugs containing opiates
Derived from opium these are: codeine phosphate, Palfium, Doloxene, Doloxene CO (particularly dangerous with alcohol or

tranquillizers), Co-proxamol, Distalgesic/Paxalgesic, DF118 and
Co-dydramol* ('Paramol').

Note Caffeine is a mild stimulant often added to painkillers (such
as Propain*, Solpadeine*, Syndol* and Doloxene CO) *but it does
not relieve pain*. On the contrary, research shows that caffeine
both increases sensitivity to pain and irritates the gut. Another
problem with caffeine is that it can cause headaches, either if you
take too much of it or if you stop taking it.

Non-steroidal anti-inflammatories (or NSAIDs)

These include aspirin, and are widely used for the relief of back
pain. They work locally at the site of injury or inflammation to
reduce enzyme activity there. They don't carry the risks of *steroids*
(see below) but can cause ulcers and can seriously aggravate
asthma. Examples of NSAIDs are *ibuprofen** (better known as
'Nurofen' and 'Brufen'), *diclofenac* (brand names are 'Voltarol' and
'Voltarol Retard'), *indomethacin* ('Indocid', 'Mobilan'), *mefenamic
acid* ('Ponstan'), *naproxen* ('Naprosyn') and *piroxicam* ('Feldene').
Gels, for local application, are Oruvail*, Ibuleve* and Proflex*.

Muscle relaxants

These are basically tranquillizers – for example *diazepam* – which
have a relaxing effect on your muscles. To relax muscle spasm
similar doses are used as for treating anxiety but they are very
addictive and should only be given short term. Tranquillizers like
diazepam work as a brain sedative even at low doses, which
means they may lead to loss of concentration and memory. This is
important to know for anyone operating machinery, for example.

Anti-depressants

These, for example *amitriptyline,* are prescribed to counteract the
depressing effects of continuous pain. Like all drugs which affect
the brain (*psychoactive drugs*) these have many unwelcome
side-effects. Anti-depressants alone also do nothing to tackle the
feelings which may be lurking below the surface of people with
long-term pain (for example, of rage and frustration).

Anabolic steroids

These are currently being researched to see if they can help
break down scar tissue.

**Indicates drugs available in some countries over the counter in
your local pharmacy without a doctor's prescription .*

Conventional further tests for back pain

To help doctors in their diagnosis – particularly if your pain is severe, prolonged or coming back more and more often – they may ask for any or all of the following further tests to be carried out.

- *Laboratory blood tests* These check the balance of your blood and look for signs of *inflammatory disease* – see Chapter 3.
- *X-rays* X-rays show changes within bones and are useful for screening out major problems with the bones, tumours or infection. Advanced *ankylosing spondylitis* will also show up on x-ray, as will changes to do with an ageing spine.

The 'pros' and 'cons' of spinal x-rays

For
- They are a quick way to check for damage or disease in the spine.
- The test itself does not cause any pain (except that of lying on a hard table with a bad back.)

Against
- The information gained is poor. The majority of back pain is caused by injuries to the soft tissues – for example, to the muscles, ligaments, discs and cartilage – and these do not show up on x-rays.
- The risk of inaccuracy is high. Repeated studies to see whether recognized experts could find fractures, gallstones, kidney stones or cancerous growths have shown a surprisingly high level of inaccuracy. The error rate for the detection of cancers normally visible on x-rays, for example, was 20–50 per cent.
- The risks to health are high. Even a small amount of radiation can do severe damage to your body. The risk increases the longer and the more often you are exposed to x-rays. Pregnant women, children and the breast area

---

of adolescent girls are particularly sensitive to radiation's known cancer-causing effects.

Summary

The risks, the cost and the limited usefulness of the information gained from x-rays mean that doctors are now sending fewer people to have them. If you have been refused an x-ray it is probably because your doctor is fairly certain that neither a fracture nor a disease is the cause of your problem.

Therapies your doctor may offer you

After your doctor has arrived at an accurate diagnosis of your condition the following are the sort of non-drug therapies you are likely to be offered.

Physiotherapy

In Britain this is normally the only manual ('hands-on') therapy on offer in state-funded medicine. Physiotherapists (physical therapists) have three to four years of state-regulated training which includes working in hospitals. Many train in specialist areas on top of this. Your initial appointment will be similar to the one with the doctor but probably in more detail. What a physiotherapist will offer you to help your back can vary enormously, and could include any of the following:

- first aid including heat treatment or ice packs
- advice on self-help in the home and at work
- exercises (one of the physiotherapist's main beliefs is that your body can often correct itself if the right exercises are given)
- massage – not just for relaxation but for specific effects (see Chapter 7, p. 93)
- joint articulation (moving joints in a controlled way to

diagnose problems or to increase their range of movement)

- *joint 'manipulation'* – although this does not usually include the short, sharp movements such as the 'high velocity thrust' employed by chiropractors as their main technique. All physiotherapists learn the so-called 'Maitlands Mobilization', which uses a graded series of hand pressures to stretch and move joints within a comfortable range. This eases the 'bind' of tight muscles, adhesions, scarred joint capsules and so on. Like massage, it also improves the exchange of body fluids in and out of the joints.

Electronic machines

These are often used to save time in busy physiotherapy departments, or in the belief that they are superior to well-trained hands. Machines in common use are:

Utrasound This creates a high-pitched sound by passing electricity through a crystal located inside the metal head of the instrument, which then glides across your skin. It is painless and soundless. Though research so far has shown inconclusive results for it, ultrasound seems to speed up healing by causing cells to vibrate in sympathy with the sound waves applied to them. It certainly can be useful when damaged soft tissues are too tender to touch but can worsen your condition if bleeding is still going on.

Interferential therapy This uses two currents set up to 'interfere' with each other to produce a tingling sensation in the patient. The currents are applied via suckers or moist sponges and can give short-term pain relief. Its long-term value is not clear.

Short wave diathermy This uses electromagnetic waves to speed up healing, whether in fractures which are slow to repair or in damaged soft tissues. As no heat is produced by the modern pulsed-dose machines they can be used safely.

TENS machines TENS stands for transcutaneous (across the skin) electrical nerve stimulation, and uses our knowledge of the gate theory of pain (see box, p. 28) to achieve its effect. It is used in pain clinics throughout the world with people in severe and often chronic pain. An electrical current is passed between two electrodes strapped to the skin at the most painful points. The stream of tingling impulses blocks the feeling of pain, though it does not tackle the cause of it.

Research into TENS

In 1976 both the American *Journal of Chinese Medicine* and the publication *Pain* reported the results of two separate studies comparing TENS with acupuncture in the treatment of low back and sciatic pain. TENS was found to be of short-term help in half the patients but acupuncture helped significantly more people and for longer. The advantage of TENS is that it can be used under paramedical supervision whereas acupuncture needs a qualified practitioner.

Hydrotherapy

This is a therapy based on the healing properties of water and involves anything from drinking it to being immersed in it. In physiotherapy it usually means you get into the water, often with the practitioner, who then treats you or guides your movements. Hydrotherapy is an ancient method of natural healing finding rapid acceptance by many doctors, though it is still 'alternative' to many. The principle behind it is simple: water supports much of your weight thus taking pressure off your spine. A modern study by rheumatologists published in 1992 compared three different types of hydrotherapy used in the treatment of low back pain and found that all three groups needed significantly lower doses of painkillers than the untreated group, even a whole year later.

Traction

This literally means 'pulling'. It can be done manually, which people often enjoy, or with contraptions looking like instruments of torture the sufferer is strapped into. The object is to stretch the tissues and take pressure off the discs. Mechanical traction is applied in hospital to people in extreme pain from nerve-root pressure. It is less popular because you are not allowed out to perform normal bodily functions, and the enforced bed rest causes many problems, not least constipation. The benefits of strong traction are hotly disputed among the experts, but there are undoubtedly people who have been greatly helped by it. (See pp. 47–8 for self-help traction.)

Other conventional options

- *Chiropody* Chiropodists treat feet and a good chiropodist can make all the difference to the way you walk, which might have been the cause of your back pain in the first place.
- *Dentistry* Dentistry can help a great deal if your 'bite' or jaw joint is upsetting your back. Remind your doctor if your problems started after heavy or lengthy dental work, particularly if your symptoms include face, head, neck or shoulder pains.
- *Orthotics* This is the branch of medicine that provides custom-made mechanical aids such as corsets, limbs, shoe-lifts and other appliances. If you suffer from a deformity that might be leading to back pain over a period of years you could be referred to a hospital department that specializes in fitting such aids. An offshoot is:
- *Podiatry* This is the art of balancing the way your feet contact the ground using individually made shoe-inlays. Although the idea is old, podiatry is a relatively new development from America. The therapy often uses sophisticated measuring equipment and ultra-

modern materials to make the inlays. It can be rather expensive as a result. Osteopaths and chiropractors sometimes have access to good reasonably priced podiatrists.

- *Pain clinics* Pain clinics are becoming common now in many parts of the world for the specialist management and treatment of both acute and chronic pain. Offering a wide range of options, including those described in this book under both conventional and unconventional headings, the better ones are becoming excellent examples of integrated or 'holistic' medicine in effective practice.

- *Rehabilitation centres* As the name implies 'rehab centres', as medics like to call them, specialize in returning you to full fitness after accident, trauma or operation. They concentrate on teaching you how to work with any aids you may have been fitted with (see 'orthotics') and toning up your muscles to cope.

Seeing a specialist

You may be one of the unlucky people who is not helped by anything your doctor or therapist can do. If nothing has helped, further investigations are needed after blood tests and x-rays have been done, or your symptoms do not fit into any recognizable pattern, your doctor is likely to turn to any one of the following specialists (a specialist is a more highly trained and experienced doctor with a special interest and in-depth knowledge of your type of problem). Because back pain is such an enormous field there are several kinds of specialist; those mentioned are the main ones.

- *Rheumatologists* They diagnose and treat people with inflammatory disorders such as *rheumatoid arthritis* and *ankylosing spondylitis* – see Chapter 3.

- *Neurologists* They diagnose and treat problems to do with the nervous system, which includes the brain.
- *Orthopaedic consultants* They diagnose and treat any problem to do with the skeletal system and everything that makes it move.
- *Psychologists* They help treat problems of the mind that can contribute to symptoms like back pain.
- *Surgeons* If, in extreme cases, surgery is considered necessary there are two sorts of surgeons you are likely to be referred to. They are:
  - *neurosurgeons* (they operate on the skull and the spinal column and their contents: for back pain this includes operations to relieve compression on a nerve caused by a damaged disc, enlarged facet joint or bony spur)
  - *orthopaedic surgeons* (they do more 'repositioning' work on, for example, fractures, deformities, joint replacements and soft tissues)

What a specialist does

A specialist will check through your whole medical history to date, will take a case history and examine you all over again. Sometimes further x-rays might be useful or, if plain x-rays do not give enough information, one of the latest forms of *scans* might be considered. Scans use different forms of energy, ranging from sound to magnetic energy, to make more detailed pictures of your painful tissues. Different types of scans gather different types of information. All of them use expensive equipment and will probably involve you in a trip to a big medical centre.

The following is a guide to the scans you might be offered. (They are covered in detail because a natural therapist might refer you for one, too, if your problem warrants it.)

CT (or CAT) scan

This uses minimal doses of x-rays (one second for the whole head) and a scanning device which whizzes around recording the different thicknesses of tissues and translating them on to film. This can find and make an image of a thin layer of your body where the tissues show signs of injury. One specialist comparing the two methods said that 'reading an x-ray is like trying to see through the whole bible at once, whereas CAT scans allow us to read one page at a time'.

MRI (magnetic resonance imaging) scan

This has a similar purpose to a CAT scan but uses very powerful electromagnets instead of x-rays. There are no known ill-effects from using strong magnets (unless you wear a pacemaker!) and they can even help .

Scans: the good and bad news

Both CT and MRI scans are used when x-rays do not give enough useful information. The good news is that both are potentially less harmful, and both allow the all-important soft tissues to be seen. Both have made many operations unnecessary, especially 'exploratory operations' done 'just to have a look inside'. Even many operations which *would* have looked like a good idea after thorough old-fashioned methods of diagnosis have been shown to be pointless after such scans.

The bad news is that scanning involves you in having to lie very still in a very confined space surrounded by huge machines while the operator disappears off into another room and talks to you through a microphone from behind a glass window. In the case of a CT scan this may be for only a few minutes but for a detailed spinal MRI scan the process can last 45 minutes.

Ultrasound scan

This is a quick and painless means of looking deep into your spine using sound waves too high to be picked up by the human ear. The amount of 'echo' produced by pointing the source of the sound waves at human tissues varies, and so a picture can be formed.

Myelogram

Sometimes called *'radiculography'* because it looks at nerve roots (think of 'radishes'), this is an uncomfortable test lasting about half an hour. It uses x-rays and a dye injected into the spinal canal and allowed to spread around the nerve roots and spinal cord. The x-ray films show which nerves are most affected and allow a surgeon to pinpoint where to operate. The dyes used, particularly the older oil-based ones, have had a mixed safety record – but as one experienced neurosurgeon put it: 'A myelogram is still safer than a scalpel'. The technique is normally only used if surgery is being considered, and is sometimes used together with the next test to localize the site of the problem even more accurately.

Electromyography

This is like checking for faulty wiring between the spinal cord and the muscles. Fine needles are inserted into muscles, usually in your leg, calf or foot, because they are the ones most commonly affected by disc disease. The electrical activity of individual muscle groups is then measured when your spine is at rest or moving. If the response of a muscle group is not as good as it should be this points the blame back at the exact nerve roots concerned.

Treatments a specialist might offer

There is a barrage of yet further tests available if the cause of your problem remains a mystery. But this is also the point at which you might look into natural therapies, if you haven't done so before, because from this point on, specialist conventional treatment tends to go down the route of ever more high-technology and stronger drugs.

For example, a specialist may recommend any of the treatments outlined before (physiotherapy, medication and so on) or might recommend injections or surgery.

Injections used to treat back pain

Facet joint injections These usually contain a steroid and an anaesthetic. They are painful when given but can give short-term relief lasting from a few hours up to several months in cases of severe arthritics (for whom education on the use of their backs has been too little too late). It is also given in the general physician's surgery to 'normal' back pain sufferers, sometimes into many of the facet joints at the same time, merely to treat the pain.

Steroid injections These are given for back pain into the facet joints (see above), other inflamed joints that could be affecting your back, sprained ligaments (if it is possible to get at them: some run very deep), and muscles – combined with cooling spray and stretching if there are 'trigger points' within the muscle. (A trigger point is a point that causes pain in another area altogether if you press it. 'Trigger point therapy' can easily be done without the injections by anyone trained to use their hands and a can of cold spray – for example, your doctor, a physiotherapist or a natural therapist.) The effectiveness of steroid injections in pain relief seems to increase the more practised the person is doing them. If you do opt for this treatment find someone who does them all the time.

Warning Repeated steroid injections are known to cause weakening of the bones, ligaments and muscle attachments around the site of the injections. This is no help to someone trying to strengthen their back. Injections are no substitute for taking positive steps to help yourself first (see chapter 4 on self-help). A good doctor should tell you the same thing.

Sclerosant injections (known as 'prolotherapy' in the USA) These are injections to 'sclerose' or harden and tighten ligaments that have become too lax and floppy. Sclerosant injections are mostly performed by private orthopaedic physicians in the UK, and in the USA by medically trained osteopaths. The injections contain an irritant solution which causes extra fibrous tissue to form around the site of injection. It is quick (about 15 minutes) but painful, and can be done under a mild anaesthetic such as 'gas and air'. You will have to wait about eight weeks before you feel better as it takes that time for the tissues to build up with weekly injections. There is no guarantee that it will work for you long term but some people have been fine for many years afterwards.

Epidural injections These are an injection of anaesthetic and steroid into the spinal canal to numb pain from disc protrusions. A milder anaesthetic is used than during childbirth and the steroid is added as an anti-inflammatory. The injection is also lower down, through the base of the spine. Epidural injections are given to people with 'nerve root signs' – for example, sciatica, back pain, muscle-wasting and sluggish lower leg reflexes – who have not responded to painkillers, rest, massage, manipulation, exercise or traction. It allows you to 'play for time' and let your body break down the damaged disc by itself while you put off plaster jackets, prolonged traction, myelography and surgery. Most disc problems, however, turn out not to be protrusions and heal in time.

Chemonucleolysis If you come from a hot country you will know that the papaya fruit is an excellent aid to digestion. One of the substances the papaya contains is an enzyme which will digest the soft nucleus of discs if injected into them. The process is called *chemonucleolysis*. The consultant doing the injecting may refer to a *myelogram* and will certainly have an x-ray monitor running in order to place the needle correctly. After the injection you may be very sore for a time as this nasty substance can leak on to sensitive areas. *Chemonucleolysis* will shrink a bulging disc permanently but can also cause severe disc collapse, putting more pressure on surrounding joints. It is also useless for severe protrusions with floating disc particles around them. In the unlikely event that this is what you have you will probably be recommended surgery.

Surgery for back pain

Surgery is not normally performed for back pain alone. You would have to have severe leg or arm pain too before a surgeon would normally consider putting you under the knife. If you have been correctly selected for surgery the chances are that you will be helped. Not everybody is completely pain free afterwards, though, and you will still have to work at improving the state of your back.

If you are in need of disc surgery be reassured that this is not quite the major event it used to be. Many operations are now done 'blind' through tiny *incisions* (cuts in the skin) using a binocular microscope and continuous x-rays to guide the surgical instruments.

After the operation you should notice a gradual improvement in your nerve root symptoms over a period of weeks. But don't forget that they might not have moved properly for years and they need to be able to slide at least 0.75cm to be comfortable when, for example, you stretch one leg out in front of you.

Don't forget also that you had a damaged back in the first place, and this still needs sorting out. Take the surgeon's advice. If necessary see someone with experience in *back rehabilitation* (getting your back fit for normal life after an injury or operation). This could mean:

- seeing a physiotherapist
- attending a 'back school', if your hospital has one
- seeing an osteopath or a chiropractor (either of these natural therapists have much to offer in ironing out the problems that led to the need for surgery in the first place, as well as the after-effects of the operation itself)
- working very gradually and gently with an *experienced* gym instructor or sports therapist

Surgery should be a last resort as a cure for back pain because results cannot be guaranteed and because it is still the most invasive treatment available. This means that there are the usual risks linked with any operation, such as:

- reaction to anaesthetics
- chest infection
- blood clots
- infection of the wound
- *haemorrhage* (sudden and severe blood loss, very occasionally needing a blood transfusion)

In the case of *spinal surgery* there are some special risks.

- *Spinal nerve or spinal cord damage* (This is rare but does lead to some form of paralysis in one out of every 5,000 operations.)
- *Death* (The mortality rate is very low – statistically, about a three in a thousand chance during or as a result of the operation – and if it happens it is usually the result of severe damage to the spinal cord or from

a blood clot lodging in the lungs. This is more likely in *major* operations.)

If you have fears talk them through with your surgeon (*and* your doctor if you wish) and don't go ahead until you feel satisfied that the possible benefits outweigh the risks. A good surgeon will back you all the way in your cautious approach.

It's time now to take a look at the 'gentle alternatives' to drugs and surgery for back pain.

CHAPTER 6

The natural therapies and back pain

Introducing the 'gentle alternatives'

By and large the so-called 'gentle' approaches to back pain cover treatment by what is being called 'alternative' or 'complementary medicine' and what this series is calling simply 'natural medicine'. Another term for it, because its ideas and concepts do not generally fit into the accepted norms of 'orthodox' or conventional medicine, is 'unorthodox' or 'unconventional' medicine.

In June 1993 the British Medical Association (BMA) published a landmark report on what *it* called 'non-conventional medicine' and in this report, which completely reversed an earlier report, the BMA conceded that the natural therapies were not only here to stay but that they had something to offer and would and should become more widely available, even to patients of conventional Western medical doctors.

Various similar studies, including ones on specific therapies, had been done earlier by a number of other organizations, and had showed that what the BMA said should happen was in fact already happening. Literally millions of appointments are made each year with natural therapists around the world. With consumer surveys showing patient satisfaction levels consistently high – between 60 and 80 per cent – the BMA was really only bowing to the inevitable.

But the report was still a landmark because it was one of the first official acknowledgements from a stronghold of conventional medical opinion that natural medicine was here to stay, and this has particular importance for sufferers from back pain.

In Britain both osteopathy and chiropractic – two of the most effective natural therapies for back pain – have now been established by Act of Parliament and will shortly have their own governing bodies recognized by the state.

In the case of chiropractic this recognition followed a two-year study comparing chiropractic with hospital outpatient treatment on some 750 people with severe or chronic back pain. This study, published in the *British Medical Journal* in 1990, showed that patients treated by chiropractors did so well, both immediately and especially in the long term, that introducing chiropractic into the free state national health service was recommended.

State recognition for the natural therapies is, in fact, much further advanced in many other countries than in Britain. In some states in America and in countries like Israel and South Africa, for example, complementary therapists enjoy equal status with doctors in the practice of a wide range of treatments, from homoeopathy to herbalism and naturopathy.

But what exactly are these therapies and what is it about them that appeals to people so much? What do they have in common and which, more to the point, are likely to help your bad back? Most importantly, how do you find a practitioner you can rely on and trust?

Why choose a natural therapy?

There are many very good reasons why you might choose natural therapies to treat your back pain. For example, you might:

- have been inspired by seeing someone close to you benefit from natural medicine
- have people around you who have benefited in the past from natural therapies, and keep encouraging you to try them
- have tried everything that is on offer in conventional medicine, and still be in pain
- be sensitive to the drugs used to treat back pain, or worried about their side-effects
- be the sort of person who simply prefers to use their own strengths to sort out a problem rather than masking its symptoms with drugs
- be considering surgery as a last resort to your problem, and might be quite sceptical about natural therapies as an option but still be prepared to give them a try before submitting to the knife. (There are, in fact, cases of people having had treatment by natural methods while awaiting surgery – and then finding they didn't need the surgery after all.)

Whatever brought you to this point, you are not alone. You are part of a groundswell of change which is sweeping through medicine around the world. People clearly want more from medicine than the feeling of being on a conveyor belt while someone else does their thinking for them.

Any number of surveys and reports have now shown conclusively that what people are looking for, very often, from doctors and healers are the following:

- to be seen as a 'whole' - that is, a combination of mind and spirit as well as body
- to have detailed attention given to their own account of their problem
- to have treatments that view their symptoms as useful, not things to be masked without treating their causes

- to have treatments that involve them actively in the
  healing process
- to have treatments that work without the invasion of
  cutting, burning, freezing or being irradiated and
  drugged
- to have treatments and medicines with no serious
  side-effects
- to have treatment that is cost-effective. (This seems to
  be one very good reason why many doctors and most
  governments are also now showing an interest.)

Conventional medicine, for all its good works and
breath-taking technology, often fails to provide one or
more of the above. So starts the trail of discovery that
growing numbers of people are now setting off upon in
the search for gentle, safe and effective medicine.

'What will my doctor say?'

One of the things that puts many people off seeking help
'outside the system' is fear of what their doctor will say,
and the fear that he will be less ready to help if the
patient has 'gone behind his back'. But this should not be
a worry.

It is always best to take your doctor into your confidence if you can – and a good one will always understand and support you – but it is *your* body, mind and
spirit that are at stake not your doctor's. And if your
doctor is one of those who doesn't understand, and
won't support you, you are probably better off going to
someone else anyway.

The chances are, though, your doctor may know as
little as you about the 'alternative' approaches you're
interested in. The rest of this chapter is all about the
background to these 'natural' approaches, to help you
not only understand better what you might be getting

into, but also explain it to your doctor. But a word of encouragement first.

Although you may be nervous of talking to your doctor about your wish to try natural therapies you may be pleasantly surprised if you are brave. Many of the methods of treating back pain conventionally are risky, and many of the rest just don't work for everybody. Doctors get tired of the situation, too, as they enjoy seeing people get better.

Doctors are also affected by the present global mood change. Those with an interest in natural therapies will have their ear to the ground, and may be able to recommend a good local practitioner for you. More and more doctors *are* recommending natural therapists, and this practice will clearly grow as more state-recognized registers are formed. Also, increasing numbers of doctors visit natural therapists themselves, and still more are interested in learning about them.

What are natural therapies and what do they have in common?

At first glance many natural therapies can seem very different from each other. Some are full of basic and obvious common sense, while others might appear quite mysterious. Some take years to learn, while the basics of others can be picked up in a matter of weeks. Some, like herbalism, are based on familiar Western ideas, while others, like acupuncture, are built on Eastern concepts that Western science finds hard to accept.

In its 1993 report the BMA stated that the natural therapies were based on a mixture of styles and techniques with nothing in common at all. In fact it couldn't have been more wrong. For, far from working within a hopeless muddle of ideas, the natural therapies all hold very much to the following principles.

- The human body has a natural tendency and ability to heal itself.
- The human body is more than the sum of its moving parts – each has a mind and 'spirit' (or 'soul') of its own, and the health of each of these aspects can make a difference to the course of a person's recovery.
- 'No man is an island' – so environmental and social factors can have as much of an impact on a person's health as can physical or psychological ones.
- Treating causes is more important than treating symptoms. While every therapist aims to help a person free themselves of symptoms, their duty is to find and treat the root causes if possible, so that symptoms do not reappear in a more serious form later on.
- Every person is unique, and cannot be treated in exactly the same way as every other person with the same condition. Natural therapists treat people, not symptoms or conditions.
- True healing has to happen *within* the 'patient', and this can only happen when patients take responsibility for their health. This does not mean they are to be 'blamed' for all that has gone before, or that they are being punished for neglecting themselves. But good health is not just a matter of finding a 'quick fix'. Problems happen for a reason and if you join in the search for the answers you will learn far more than if you just hand the job over to the therapist.

Natural therapies useful in the treatment of back pain

Natural therapies fall roughly into two camps, treating either the mind and emotions or the body – but always looking at both. All of them have something to offer you, the back pain sufferer, if used at the right time.

Therapies that treat the body are 'physical therapies'. These tend to look for mechanical imbalances and help restore these to a comfortable state. This is your most obvious 'first port of call' in trying to heal your back. These therapies are dealt with in Chapter 7.

Therapies that treat your mind and emotions are 'psychological therapies'. These tend to look for emotional or mental imbalances and aim to help you regain your sense of inner calm. These are explained in Chapter 8.

If you look at any of these therapies more closely, though, you will see that all of them treat all of you. Psychotherapy, for example, might help you see your life situation quite differently, and the relief can feel very physical. On the other hand, a really good massage therapist can help you reach a state of deep mental relaxation whilst basically kneading muscles.

There is also a group of therapies which are 'systems of medicine'. Examples are acupuncture and homoeopathy. These aim to shift energy rather than joints or attitudes. Such therapies fall very firmly between the previous two stools and they are covered in Chapter 9.

It is not just *what* the therapies do that matters, however, but also *how* the therapist practises them. A practitioner should not only be well qualified but should also be wholehearted about trying to help the *whole* of you. This kind of approach to health has come to be called 'holistic' (after the Greek word *holos*, meaning 'whole'). Indeed the better doctors now increasingly follow this principle – so much so that in some countries, such as America and Britain, they have their own organizations to foster and promote it (see Appendix A).

If at first you don't succeed

Whatever your situation you cannot help but be guided in your choice of therapy by your preferences, fears, prejudices and by whoever has advised you. These influences will not always lead you to the right place – first time – but they will open a door for you.

If you have made a mistake in your choice be clear that no responsible natural therapist should keep you trailing along for more than two or three treatments without both of you feeling reasonably sure that you are on the right road. Good therapists will care more about your welfare than about their bank balance and will gladly suggest someone more suitable for you. This should not be seen as a sign of failure of either the therapy or the practitioner. No one should guarantee to cure your problem, and no one can do more than their best.

One of the most important aspects of any health problem, including back pain, is that you are dedicated to getting better. In this sense your input is more important than anybody else's.

Summary

If you are under the care of medical staff for your back pain at the moment it is only courteous to let them know of your plans to try natural therapies. If you get a negative reaction, don't be put off! Doctors are human, too, and may remember scare stories more readily than success stories. If you get good results from using a natural therapist, do tell your doctor – it helps to redress the balance.

To find the approach which suits you best, read the next three chapters on the different natural therapies with a good track record of dealing with back pain. The last chapter will then help you find a therapist you can rely on and trust.

CHAPTER 7

Treating your body

Physical therapies that work

The most commonly used therapies in the treatment of back pain are the 'hands-on' ones listed below. Therapies in **bold** print are well researched, tried and tested and covered in detail in this chapter. The remaining therapies may be effective – and certainly that is their claim – but the proof is not really there in convincing enough detail yet. Information on all of them is available from the national umbrella organizations for the natural therapies listed in Appendix A. Physical therapies recommended for back pain are:

- **Alexander Technique***
- **applied kinesiology** – Touch for Help*
- aromatherapy*
- **chiropractic**
- Feldenkrais method*
- Heller work
- **massage***
- neuromuscular technique
- **osteopathy (and cranial osteopathy)**
- qi-gong*
- rolfing
- t'ai chi ch'uan*
- **yoga***

Therapies you can do yourself with training

The techniques used in these therapies all contain a lot of overlap. This is partly because many of them grew out of common ground many thousands of years ago (we know this from surviving cave drawings, hieroglyphs and ancient texts). But it is also because, despite healthy competition between many therapies, new developments are often shared between them as they happen and compatible approaches adopted. However there are some important differences in their approaches.

Alexander Technique

Named after the Australian actor F. Matthias Alexander who devised the technique early this century, the Alexander Technique is learning and therapy rolled into one. Alexander showed that bad postural habits we develop as we get older can have an important effect on our health but that these can be corrected with 're-education' of our bodies. To emphasize this Alexander therapists are called 'teachers' rather than therapists and the technique is something you must first learn by taking lessons. But it does not take many – between four and six on average – and once learned you can easily then do the technique for yourself.

For the approach to be effective, though, you have to be prepared to change the whole way you move and think. Early lessons involve very gentle hands-on therapy in which you allow the therapist to apply gentle releasing techniques to tight areas. But later lessons mean relearning everything; from the way you walk and run to how you breathe and write. Alexander teachers say the technique is about 'being' in a state of balance with minimum effort, not just about how you move. But once you start doing it you should feel tense mental habits ebbing away with the physical ones. (*See figure 6.*)

Use of the technique has grown hugely in the last few

years. In Britain, for example, many hospitals now have it in their pain clinics and all British music colleges offer it as a preventive therapy for their students. In fact the technique seems to have been adopted wholesale by actors, dancers and artistes of many sorts who have found it enhances and extends their performing abilities.

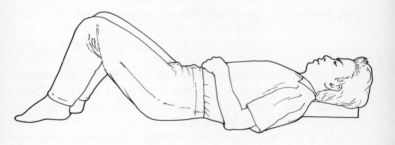

Fig 6. An Alexander Technique relaxation exercise

Applied kinesiology

This is a system of diagnosis and treatment known loosely as 'muscle-testing'. It grew out of a self-help energy-balancing method originally developed by American chiropractors after the Second World War. Originally called 'Touch for Health', 'AK', as it is known for short, is practised mainly by osteopaths and chiropractors although Russian neurologists have recently been learning it from British teachers for use in hospitals there.

The principle behind AK is that 'energy pathways', or *meridians*, in the body (see 'Acupuncture' Chapter 9) are thought to be linked to different muscles. These can be individually tested for strength and this gives the practitioner subtle information about a person's energy levels and nervous system.

Practitioners also believe that any muscle that tests 'strong' normally will test 'weak' with something that places particular stress on a person's system and, equally, a muscle that tests 'weak' in the first place will test 'strong' when the deficiency is put right.

So, for instance, a person with a sensitivity to sugar will test 'weak' if a tiny pinch of sugar is placed on the tip of the tongue and the previously strong muscle is re-tested. AK is therefore used to diagnose food and other chemical sensitivities and intolerances. Equally, if someone is deficient in, say, zinc, placing the right amount of zinc on their tongue will strengthen a previously weak muscle. This system is therefore used to correct nutritional imbalances in the body.

AK is a fairly complicated system that takes time to learn. It borrows from every branch of medicine and uses your body as a sort of 'bio-computer' that can answer its own questions. It needs considerable knowledge to be applied effectively and can be abused, and unfortunately is, by those with more enthusiasm than skill. In the right hands, though, it has been used successfully to help many people with back problems who could not be healed by other methods.

Chiropractic

This is a system of diagnosis and treatment developed in America at the end of the last century that relates your body's level of comfort to how well its parts are moving – and in particular whether the spinal nerves are able to work freely.

Chiropractors use x-rays to help them make their initial diagnosis (for the pros and cons of x-rays see pp. 67–8) and on to this they add what they observe in their detailed and subtle physical examination. From this they decide which *facet joints* of the spine to manipulate.

Chiropractors do treat and take into account all the other parts of the body but they have become best known for their skill in treating spinal problems. The techniques they use tend to involve short, sharp thrusts directly on to 'stuck' joints. This usually results in a 'clicking' noise as the joint concerned becomes 'freed'. It may sound loud if done in your neck but the movement itself is tiny. Your spinal joints may well be manipulated in this way several times a week and then at longer intervals until your problem resolves.

From its beginnings in America chiropractic is now the most established of the natural therapies with more practitioners around the world than any other therapy. In the USA alone, for example, there are more than 30,000 practitioners with a status almost the equal of conventional medical doctors, though they don't yet have automatic access to the full range of hospital facilities. In Britain, where almost 600 chiropractors account for a total of 75,000 treatments a week, they became established by special Act of Parliament in 1994 and will have their own state-recognized governing body by about 1996.

Massage

Based on the natural reaction of wanting to hold or rub a painful area, massage is probably among the very earliest of the manual healing arts known to humankind. It has developed into a highly skilled practice since those days, of course, and research galore now confirms the beneficial effects that have probably always been felt – as well as some that may not have been realized.

Direct or 'mechanical' effects

- friction warming
- pumping circulation
- stretching soft tissue
- breaking down scar tissue
- breaking down adhesions
- improved tissue *permeability* (this means pores in the tissues open up better, allowing wastes out and fresh blood in quicker)
- opening micro-circulation (this means blood flow in the tissues is increased by blood vessels becoming wider from the effects of pressure)
- release of enzymes (these are needed to speed up all bodily chemical reactions)
- improved tissue *elasticity* (or 'stretchiness', achieved by the combination of all massage movements)

Indirect or 'reflex' effects

- relaxation (through local loosening of tight tissues, general calming throughout the body and the massage of specific points which induce relaxation)
- pain reduction (by improving local drainage of painful waste products like *lactic acid*, by stretching muscles and muscle fascia to reduce 'body splinting', and by stimulating pain-killing substance – *endorphin* – release)
- opening micro-circulation (this time through nerve reflexes, with only light pressure)
- balancing the *autonomic nervous system* (responsible for non-voluntary muscular movements like heartbeats and digestion)

Massage can also be used to reduce high blood pressure and normalize bowel function in constipation. This all matters to backs because problems in other areas will overload the spinal cord, resulting in muscle spasm around the spine.

Therapeutic massage might be less of a 'quick fix' than joint manipulation but for some people it may be the right pace of change. However if you have back pain that improves but does not go away after a few massages you are more likely to need treatment by one of the other therapies covered in this chapter, particularly chiropractic, cranial osteopathy or osteopathy. They are generally more useful in clearing long-standing and severe back pain.

Osteopathy

Osteopathy, like chiropractic, aims to restore comfortable working function to areas of the body such as backs that are 'stuck'. Unlike chiropractors, though, osteopaths rarely use x-rays and their emphasis is more on the soft tissues.

It is another therapy developed by an American pioneer at the end of the last century, but some osteopaths claim osteopathy is not a technique so much as a philosophy of mind and movement. In other words, the comfort and health of the human body depends on healthy movement. So where there is stagnation of movement – whether of a joint, a body fluid or an attitude – there is 'dis-ease', and therefore the potential for disease itself.

As in chiropractic, an osteopathic case history and physical examination is detailed and refined and the techniques vary enormously. You may be massaged firmly and stretched rhythmically before any joint manipulation is done at all – this is known as 'soft tissue manipulation' – and if a spinal joint is to be manipulated it is more likely to be done using 'levers' within the body to stretch a joint until it frees rather than applying vigorous pressure to a facet joint itself.

In America, where it began, all osteopaths are medical doctors. Elsewhere, though, the situation is the complete opposite. Osteopaths are mostly non-medical specialists who have trained in osteopathy (and some also in natur-opathy) as a separate skill. In Britain there are now more than 2,000 osteopaths trained in this way giving around 100,000 treatments a week.

Cranial osteopathy

Cranial osteopathy is a well-established extension of osteopathy effective in many cases of back pain. Cranial osteopathy is not just 'cranial' (working on the skull) but rather attempts to 'put the head on the spine'. In so doing it has brought about a little revolution in the way many osteopaths look at body health and movement.

It all began in the 1930s when an osteopath tried to disprove that the bones of the skull could move, even though there was enough space between the joints to allow for movement. He ended up making the important discovery that the bones of the skull, along with every other tissue in the body, seem to move in a slow rhyth-mic wave motion throughout life.

Cranial osteopaths consider that how well the tissues ebb and flow reflects how healthy they are as well as where they are held tight. By 'listening' to disturbances in the normal movement patterns they believe they can relate your symptoms to the structures that might be affected and set about correcting imbalances in tension.

It is an approach that believes in going *with* what your body is doing already rather than forcing corrections from outside. Among the gentlest of all hands-on thera-pies it can have powerful results and it is therefore important to see someone with the necessary clinical skills to judge your tissues' subtle responses safely.

Cranial osteopathy is particularly helpful in the treat-ment of babies and children who seem to respond well to its gentle approach.

Note In Britain non-osteopaths who practise cranial

osteopathy frequently call themselves 'sacro-cranial ther-apists' to get around the protection of the term 'osteopa-thy' now enjoyed by 'proper' osteopaths. But such therapists do not have the training and knowledge of osteopaths and may therefore not be as skilled or safe.

Back pain treatment and cost

Treatment by such highly skilled professionals as chiropractors and osteopaths is still largely outside the free health schemes of those countries with a free national service and so must be paid for privately.

In general osteopathic and chiropractic treatments are cost-effective for many people, particularly the self-employed, because these therapies can be quick to give relief from severe pain, allowing a swift return to work. People who take care of elderly or disabled family members, too, need to be back in action as quickly as possible as do professional carers.

For those in dire financial need, such as the unemployed and those whose backs prevent them from working, many practitioners operate a sliding scale of fees and may postpone or even waive certain payments. Established training colleges in most countries also have well-supervised teaching clinics where treatment is available at greatly reduced cost.

Yoga

Many specialists caution against yoga for back problems but research under way at a pioneering centre in Britain suggests it can be highly effective, particularly in treat-ing cases of long-term pain.

The Yoga Therapy Centre in London, set up in 1993, claims yoga can help chronic back pain by strengthening and toning back muscles and improving general mobili-ty. Patients learn special exercises created by a spinal

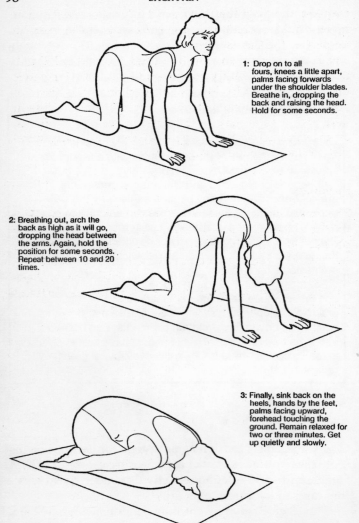

1: Drop on to all
fours, knees a little apart,
palms facing forwards
under the shoulder blades.
Breathe in, dropping the
back and raising the head.
Hold for some seconds.

2: Breathing out, arch the
back as high as it will go,
dropping the head between
the arms. Again, hold the
position for some seconds.
Repeat between 10 and 20
times.

3: Finally, sink back on the
heels, hands by the feet,
palms facing upward,
forehead touching the
ground. Remain relaxed for
two or three minutes. Get
up quietly and slowly.

Fig 7. 'The Cat' yoga exercise for backs

surgeon and yogi that they can do for themselves after supervised instruction. A good example is the exercise known as 'the Cat' (*see figure 7*).

But the centre, run by the Yoga Biomedical Trust, does not recommend yoga for acute pain nor for pelvic disorders caused by low back problems. It is also not advised for pain caused by osteoarthritis. The lesson here is that yoga may well help your back pain but see an experienced and properly qualified back pain therapist with knowledge of yoga first.

Summary

The therapies described in this chapter can be very effective at alleviating and even removing completely the physical effects of back pain. But very often, as we have seen earlier, back pain can have a cause 'beyond' the purely physical. In the next chapter we'll look at those natural therapies effective at treating the underlying psychological causes and aspects of back pain.

CHAPTER 8

Treating your mind and emotions

Psychological therapies that work

This chapter concentrates on those therapies relying on their psychological effects – that is, their effect on your mind and emotions – for tried and tested benefits in treating back problems. They are:

- psychotherapy and counselling
- hypnotherapy (and self-hypnosis*)
- meditation*
- relaxation*
- flower remedies*

Therapies you can do for yourself after some training

The link between body and mind

Few people, even professional healthcarers sometimes, seem to realize just how closely our backs and our feelings are bound up with one another. This is especially true when we are injured. It is even more true when we have been putting up with pain over a period of weeks and months.

Look at the way our feelings can affect the very way we hold ourselves. When we stand or walk, all our soft and vulnerable organs are open to the world and we ask our backs to hold us up in this exposed position whenever we face the outside world. When we're confident we 'walk tall' and feel no fear. Sometimes, though, we just don't feel proud, confident and courageous. We feel 'downcast' – so we react by letting our lower back and abdominal muscles flop and this in turn allows our torsos to slump forwards under the combined forces of gravity and negative feelings.

Another part of this sorry picture is tension and compression. Some people don't just slouch but pull their necks into their shoulders like tortoises, brace their shoulder blades down on to their backs and tighten their abdominal muscles to form a protective wall. Their spines are then caught in the crossfire between front and back.

If you add a dash of tense restricted breathing to either of these two situations, and bear in mind that our bodies are all coping with a small degree of lopsidedness at the same time, you have the recipe for back injury and pain.

How feelings cause physical injury

We know from research this century that our feelings cause actual chemical changes in our bodies. These changes can put a strain on the health of our tissues by affecting their ability to adapt. As a result the tissues either become slower or less effective at juggling the demands we put on them.

What finally tips the balance doesn't much matter. It can be nutritional stress – that is, skipping meals during a busy period or drinking lots of coffee or alcohol – a physical jolt or strain, or it could be more of the same inner tension that created the original problem.

Sometimes, often without realizing it, we are just managing – somehow. But by this stage our reserves for coping with shocks of any kind have run very low. If at times like this any extra crisis comes along (and it is amazing how often at such times not just one but a series of crises seems to crop up) our backs and necks stubbornly refuse to take any more. They lock into spasm with tremendous power – and at the very moment when we can least cope with it.

Negative responses to pain

Pain, as we all know, makes us feel depressed and fed up. These 'negative responses' are useful at first because we have to be dissatisfied with something to the point of wanting to change it before we actually do something about it. Being caught in a vice of pain will eventually stop you in your tracks, and there is always a useful lesson to be learnt from events like this.

Once you are in pain it is very tempting to become angry. But this only makes matters worse. To feel anger at the inconvenience, the injustice or simply the sheer agony is quite normal. Unfortunately this increases the levels of adrenalin pumped into your blood, making you tense up even more.

Anger can sometimes be a cover-up for fear. You might be afraid that your pain has a serious cause, or that it will go on forever. Fear is part of the body's automatic and instinctive 'fight or flight' response system. But this also increases adrenalin levels in your body.

Chronic (long-term) pain and depression

Being frightened and angry takes a lot of energy, and energy is usually something in short supply when we are in pain. That's why people during a long spell of pain lapse into a state of depression. They are emotionally and mentally exhausted. But the depression is really only the surface veil across many layers of problems, all of which need to be tackled for a cure to happen effectively.

The very smallest doses of anti-depressants *can* be helpful in chronic persistent pain and the side-effects are few but most natural therapists agree that giving people continuous drugs to lift depression is not the answer. In the long run this kind of drug-only treatment allows you to 'soldier on' – but with the real underlying causes of your problem unsolved, and sometimes even with extra ones thrown in from the effects of the medication itself (see box on 'Drugs for back pain' in Chapter 5, pp. 65–6).

Helping your back pain by helping your mind

If you feel that the pain in your back may be the result of your mental or emotional state you need to look at the physical and psychological patterns that lie behind the behaviour that is damaging to your health. You will probably need to start teaching your mind as well as your body to work in a more relaxed and balanced way. These tasks can take a lot of time and patience but you may be surprised at the rewards that follow.

Signs that back pain may be caused by emotional problems

There are several clear pointers that all is not well on the emotional front.

- A history of pain that happened after a major emotional upset or a prolonged spell of minor ones.
- A strong family history of 'bad backs' without apparent physical cause. (Some people feel doomed to getting a bad back, or have been taught from early childhood that a bad back gets attention. Either way it can become ingrained into their expectation of life. Perfectly healthy children have even been known to limp to copy their ailing elders.)
- A history of back pain since being physically injured at some point. (Even though the injury has healed the

shock or feelings that went with it may still be present: that is, they have not yet been 'let go'.)

- When there is financial gain from prolonging the injury, as in industrial or accident compensation cases: some people just want to settle their claim and put the whole thing behind them while others let their pain drag on way beyond a time when any other similar injury would have healed, and all physical signs of injury have gone, simply to get more money. Such people may not always be conscious of the 'game' they're playing – or of how obvious it can be to a professional carer.

- When there is any other kind of gain from pain – for example, if it enables you to stay away from a job you don't enjoy or to avoid 'facing the music' over some relationship issue.

- When the combined efforts of all therapists fail to find a cause or solution for your pain – you may be feeling like Humpty Dumpty because no-one seems able to 'put you together again'.

Could your problem be 'all in the mind'?

Being told that a problem for which no obvious physical cause could be found is 'all in the mind' used to be quite a common comment for doctors to pass on patients with bad backs. It does not happen quite so often now but if it happens to you don't lose heart. A hands-on therapist like an osteopath may still be able to make sense of your problem. But if you are simply one of those people with back pain caused by something the human race doesn't understand yet, don't give up, no matter how maddening you find it (in this particular case homoeopathy may be worth a try – see Chapter 9 on 'energy therapies').

However if someone you trust has come to the conclusion that there must be something bothering you enough to give you a backache it might just be true.

Your pain is real enough to you and that should not be disputed by anyone.

Try going again through the list above, and see if absolutely none of it applies to you. Hardly any of us with a pain could honestly say that there was absolutely no beneficial spin-off from being in pain. But if we give enough emotional energy to keeping the pain there – because we like the 'good effects' too much (time off work, money, sympathy and so on) – we run the risk of doing ourselves serious damage.

- Recent research has shown that people in chronic pain run the risk of doing permanent damage to special nerve cells in the spinal cord (called *inhibitory interneurons*) which naturally dampen down pain.
- Our whole nervous system can actually become geared to pain, and the signals can become very difficult to switch off.
- The longer we stay in our 'cocoon' of sickness the harder it is to re-enter the 'normal world' and take on adult responsibilities again.
- Our whole social and financial support systems start to depend on our state of disability.

What to do about emotional or psychological pain

There are various ways 'in' to your body through your mind. The rest of this chapter will describe those with proven benefit in more detail. The short answer to the question of which natural therapies can affect, and therefore help, you psychologically is that they all can. What matters is not so much the therapy as your individual needs and wants. The important thing is to choose a route that appeals to you. This form of self-selection, based on your own 'natural instinct' or intuition of what will help, is probably your best guarantee that you will benefit – simply because you want to.

Psychotherapy

The first thing to get straight is that you don't have to be mad to see a psychotherapist! A psychotherapist is nothing like a psychiatrist who is a medical doctor trained in treating mental diseases, usually with drugs or sometimes by referral for surgery. A psychotherapist is someone specially trained to help untangle deep-seated human problems simply by talking them through with you. It may be in the form of short-term 'crisis therapy' or it may be a longer-term commitment between both of you until you feel better.

When you visit a psychotherapist you will no doubt talk about more than your back pain so it is most important that you see someone with whom you feel able to be open. Good psychotherapists' organizations will go to great lengths to help you find someone in your area you are happy with.

If lack of money stops you even though you want this service there are low-cost teaching centres and charitably-run clinics in some places and your doctor or a good psychotherapy association will be able to tell you about them.

Counselling

This has the same purpose as psychotherapy but may not mean exploring your mind in quite the same depth. The purpose of counselling is *not* to give you advice but support in making your own decisions. It is to find out how you honestly feel about your problem, what you want to do about it, and helping you build up the emotional strength to start putting your plans into action.

Counselling is now becoming so widely accepted, with most hospitals and health centres employing the services of at least one counsellor these days, it is no longer the unusual or slightly 'alternative' discipline it once was. In Britain, for example, counselling is a well-run and organized profession with a highly respected central association.

Hypnotherapy (and self-hypnosis)

Hypnotherapy, or hypnosis, needs a trained therapist to help you reach what is called an 'altered state of consciousness'. Despite what you may see performed by stage hypnotists on TV hypnosis does *not* mean being 'put into a trance' or controlled in any way. In the hands of a responsible and experienced practitioner you will reach a state in which you are more easily influenced by positive suggestions made by either the therapist *or yourself*.

Despite the fact not everyone is easy to hypnotize, and so hypnotherapy does not always work, this approach has a good track-record in treating pain in general, and some research has been done on hypnotherapy and back pain.

A study in 1983, for example, monitored the progress of a group of patients with chronic low back pain who were taught self-hypnosis techniques over a period of two months. All had less pain, pain for shorter lengths of time, took less medication and got to sleep more quickly than those who were not treated.

A word of caution Hypnosis has more potential for harm than many therapies and it is essential you locate a reliable and trustworthy practitioner if you are seeking help by this route. For how to find a therapist you can trust see Chapter 10.

Meditation

Also described as 'passive concentration', meditation does not have to have the mystic associations of the various Oriental religious groups that popularized it in the West in the 1960s. Research shows conclusively that what 'passive concentration' does, done properly, is calm down your body's *sympathetic nervous system*. This is the system, centred in your brain, responsible for the famous 'fight or flight' response.

Calming down your instinct to be constantly 'on guard' – which is what the sympathetic nervous system does to you whether you like it or not – reduces the amount of adrenalin you produce and this relaxes your muscles too. Various studies have shown that using 'mindful meditation' (another description for it) can improve pain levels, mood disturbances, medication levels and many other factors associated with back pain.

Meditation is best taught by trained teachers. Meditation involves learning to relax by sitting quietly somewhere comfortable, fixing your gaze on something pleasant and constant – say, a candle flame – and clearing your mind completely. Some people find it helpful to repeat a 'mantra', a word or words chosen by you or your teacher to suggest peace and calm.

'Mantra' is an Oriental term and the most famous mantras are also Oriental but they needn't be. Choose something – for example, 'blue lagoon' – that has an impact on you or, better still, is neutral for you. In other words, it helps you shut off (and out) normal brain 'chatter'.

Relaxation

The same study as the one described under hypnotherapy also found that people who were taught relaxation techniques achieved similarly good results in reducing their back pain and the amount of drugs they took.

Of course relaxation should be as natural as breathing but a surprising number of people find this essential human function almost impossible to carry out. If this is you then you may find attending a class helpful but there are plenty of things you can do for yourself first.

- Make a commitment you will give a little time each day (30 minutes will do) just for you.
- Make a pact with yourself that nothing will disturb you at this time, and set up your living space to make this possible. The clearer you are in your own mind about this the more readily those around you will respect your needs.
- Make sure you have the *energy* to relax. (This may sound odd but relaxation needs quiet concentration. If you need to sleep go to sleep: relaxation can be done another time.)
- Believe in your ability to be calm and balanced: don't hold yourself back by telling yourself (or everyone around you) what a hopelessly tense person you are. The chances are someone undermined your confidence to relax long ago and reinforcing their message won't help you.
- Believe in your *right* to relax. It is surprising how many people, particularly in Western society, still feel guilty about relaxing, as if it were somehow almost a sin. You have *your* permission to relax and don't need anyone else's.

If you would prefer to attend classes, relaxation classes are usually found at:

- local health and fitness centres
- adult education and community centres
- hospital back school and pain clinics

There are also any number of tapes and videos on the market that can help you do the same thing at home. The British Holistic Medical Association publishes audio-tapes for relaxation as part of its *Tapes for Health* series (see Appendix A for address).

Flower remedies

Flower remedies are made from specific flowers floated for several hours in bright sunshine and the resulting liquid then preserved in alcohol (actually cheap brandy). The best known are the Bach remedies – named after their 'discoverer' Dr Edward Bach, a British physician-turned-homoeopath who turned from studying bowel samples to flowers (understandably!) earlier this century – although there are now a number of 'competing' ranges, notably from California and Australia.

The aim of all flower remedies is to treat the underlying emotional disturbances (not the symptoms) that come with any sickness or pain. They can be used for self-help as well as by therapists. There are 36 Bach remedies in the original range – though others claim to have extended them since – and all you need to try them is the leaflet that comes with them outlining the different emotional states Bach believed people commonly become stuck in.

If any of them rings the right bells with you that is the remedy (or remedies if you find several bells ringing) to use. However if you find you need several consider seeing a professional. You could be getting yourself into a distressed muddle and an experienced therapist will be able to help guide you through.

There is, in fact, no reliable scientific research proving the remedies do what they claim but in the fifty or so years since their introduction they have been in regular use by literally hundreds of thousands of people around the world and most seem to swear absolutely by their efficacy. The moral is, try them and see. They certainly can't hurt and if they help you so much the better.

Summary

The 'emotional therapies' can be extremely helpful in getting to the bottom of back pain, especially if nothing else seems to clear it. This is a complex area to try and work in by yourself because you are not always the best judge of whether you have a deep-seated emotional problem. This is why the help of a professional therapist is almost always best to get you started.

On the other hand, it is important not to get too stuck in long-term psychological therapy for back pain. It is not a well-proven therapy for it and getting stuck in something on which you may come to depend can cause more harm than good. Remember that your body will respond quite quickly when you are moving in the right direction, and that there is much you can and must do for yourself. Sitting around talking about it is only one part of the therapy jigsaw.

Another part of the jigsaw is treatment you can get from the so-called 'subtle energy' therapies like acupuncture. Let's look at those next.

CHAPTER 9

'Energy' therapies that can help back pain

Treating your 'life force'

This chapter covers therapies that claim to owe their effect to the existence of invisible and often extremely subtle energies within the body that can be used to heal illnesses in the body. The list below gives those therapies with any claim to help back pain this way. Only a few, though, have proven success – the therapies shown in **bold** type – and they are described in some detail. Information about the others can be obtained through the organizations listed in Appendix A.

- **acupuncture** (and auriculotherapy)
- **acupressure (and shiatsu)**
- chakra balancing
- crystal therapy*
- **healing (and 'therapeutic touch')**
- homoeopathy*
- **magnetotherapy***
- metamorphic technique
- **reflexology*** (and **Vacuflex** therapy)
- polarity therapy
- reiki
- spinal touch

Therapies you can do for yourself with training

What is 'energy therapy'?

The idea of treatment using invisible force-fields around and within the body may seem odd at first (so odd to some that they simply refuse to think any further) but there is actually nothing odd about it. Electricity, magnetism, radio-waves, ultrasound, x-rays, radiation and microwaves are forms of energy we are perfectly familiar with but all invisible.

A good example in conventional medicine of invisible energy forces in the human body being used in treatment is the *electrocardiograph* or ECG. This is the machine that helps in diagnosing heart disease by measuring the electrical currents – the invisible electrical currents – running through our skin.

In fact, as physicists now know, we are little more than the visible end of an energy spectrum that also includes lots of invisible forms. Long before modern physics people have sensed this energy and tried to give it a name. In India they call it *prana*, in China *qi* or *chi* (pronounced 'chee') and in Japan *ki*. In the West it used to be called by its Latin description *vis medicatrix naturae* (meaning 'the healing force of nature') but nowadays people generally refer to it as just the 'life force' or 'vital force'. Whatever its name the concept remains the same and conveys most healers', and most people's, conviction that we are not just a collection of chemicals but that some sort of fundamental 'energy' lies behind everything and it is this that we mean when we speak of 'life'.

Working with and through this life force is the claim of all the so-called 'energy therapies'. Their aim is to diagnose where, and to what extent, this 'vital force' is depleted or under strain. By intervening in various ways they try to harness the body's natural tendency for self-healing to bring about a return to a normal flow of force or vital energy, and hence full health.

Acupuncture

Acupuncture is a system of medicine which, combined with herbs, has been in common practice for about 4,000 years throughout most of the Far East, especially in China, where it started. In China it has been used to treat most problems with a high degree of success (although, interestingly, much of China is now busy adopting Western methods of medicine as fast as we are incorporating their ideas).

The treatment uses very fine steel needles – so fine most people don't even feel them being inserted – to stimulate the body's subtle energy (or *chi*) at any one or more of hundreds of specific 'acupoints' situated along the 12 'meridians' or energy pathways said to run through the body (*see figure 8*).

Needles are used to *sedate* a point (calm it down) or to *tonify* it (stimulate or 'wake it up'). This is why needles sometimes get 'twiddled' or agitated during a treatment. Some acupuncturists use points located in the ears and this has its own name: *auriculotherapy*.

A modern variation is *electro-acupuncture*. This involves using very low-voltage electrical currents applied to acupuncture points from leads attached to the needles.

Another variation, although traditional this time, is the technique known as *moxibustion*. In this a gentle heat is applied to an energy point using *moxa*, a dried powdered herb (usually common mugwort). This is either attached to the needle so that the heat transfers down the needle to the energy point or it is rolled into small cones and slowly burnt over the point on top of a protective covering. The belief is that this 'draws' and 'heats' the energy making more energy available. It might sound weird but it can work very well, especially if you are in spasm. Heat going into just the right parts of your injured back can be extremely soothing.

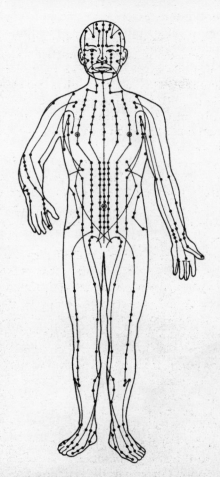

Fig 8. Acupuncture 'energy' meridians and main points

This combined practice of using acupuncture with herbs is known collectively as Traditional Chinese Medicine (TCM). The list of herbs used in Chinese medicine is vast and practitioners of TCM in the West tend to

be Chinese. Western practitioners seem to prefer to concentrate mainly on acupuncture and moxibustion.

Acupuncturists, like any other good therapist, will
begin by taking a case history and giving you a physical
examination. Since they are usually also trained in
Western medical sciences they will use conventional
methods to help them understand your problem. But
other methods they may use, such as feeling your various 'pulses' and reading your tongue, are far from conventional.

Studies around the world have shown that acupuncture can be very effective at relieving pain both in the
short and long term.

The exact way acupuncture works is still debated but
it seems the way it works to clear back pain is basically
by helping the body to produce more effective amounts
of its own painkillers, mainly *endorphins*.

Acupressure

Acupressure is a widely used and popular form of therapy which uses finger pressure (and sometimes elbow,
knee or heel pressure) on the same points of the body as
in acupuncture. This is why it is often called 'acupuncture
without needles'. Some people believe it may even have
been an earlier form of acupuncture or a variation developed for those who didn't have or didn't like needles.

The principles are the same as those of acupuncture
but most modern forms in use today were developed not
in China but Japan. The best known variation is *shiatsu*
('shiatsu' means 'finger pressure' in Japanese) but other
names you may hear are *do-in*, *jin shen* (or *shin*) and *shen
tao*. All use pressure but in different ways. Do-in, for
example, adds in breathing and exercise routines and jin
shen uses more prolonged pressure (several minutes).

The patient is lightly clothed and normally lies on a

floor mat or low table. As in acupuncture the practitioner tries to affect the level of *chi* or 'subtle energy' in the body. Back problems are said to respond very well to acupressure but in common with many natural therapies it is recommended first and foremost as a preventive measure, to keep you in a state of harmony or balance and therefore to stop problems developing.

Both acupressure and shiatsu can be very useful self-help treatments but self-help is not really recommended, or often feasible, for back pain. Neither technique is likely to help you clear pain yourself and the services of a skilled practitioner are really essential for either to have any effect at all. For a severe or long-term back problem you are probably better off going to see a doctor or someone who specializes in your sort of condition such as an osteopath or chiropractor.

Healing

Healing is the general term for the overall mending process and for those who practise the skill of mending people: doctors are, or should be, healers for example. But healing, (faith healing or spiritual healing) is also the common shorthand for therapists who claim to cure by the technique of 'laying-on-of-hands' or by transferring energy a distance by thought alone (also called 'absent healing').

There are many different ways a healer will claim to heal but most believe they are acting as a conduit or channel for a sort of universal healing energy which pours through them into the person in need of healing. Some, of course, but not all by any means, believe this power comes from God. Spiritualist healers (as opposed to spiritual healers) for example sometimes believe the healing agent is a healing entity or spirit of some sort. The basic belief however remains the same.

Believe it or not there is more evidence for the success of healing for a wide variety of conditions than any other 'natural' therapy apart from hypnosis. There is not quite so much evidence for the benefits in cases of back pain (a small study done in the 1980s showed that people with chronic low back pain who received regular weekly healing over two months were left with less pain than those who received either supportive psychotherapy or no treatment) but most healers will probably say they can help and will almost certainly want to try. Healing can, though, be highly successful at removing headaches and other pain associated with back problems.

Healing can also bring about changes that are not always physical. This means that your back pain may not go just because someone has put their hand on it. You may instead burst into tears, feel a surge of energy or a sense of having 'shed a load'. For your body at that moment your symptoms of back pain may not be top of the list of healing priorities.

Healers come from an extraordinary diversity of backgrounds and professions and it is not unusual these days to find conventional healthcare professionals, even doctors, admitting to practising healing (though sometimes only on the quiet in case they are laughed at by colleagues). They are no longer hard to find. Once you start looking for them you will find them.

Be suspicious, though, of anyone who makes huge publicity about their healing 'powers' and of anyone who pokes their nose into your life and insists you need healing. Even if it is true, you will get better results if the moment for reaching out for help is chosen by you and not by a busybody, no matter how well meaning.

In many countries claiming to heal by 'supernatural' methods is actually illegal. This is the case in most European countries and in some states in the USA (in others healers are tolerated but may not touch their patients). In America, because of the legal problems, the term more commonly used is 'therapeutic touch' and there is now a wide following among nurses and other health professionals.

By contrast the situation in Britain is the exact opposite. Anyone can heal if they feel like it and faith healing in Britain has a greater following than all the other natural therapies combined, with an estimated 30,000 practising full- or part-time healers at the last count. Doctors are also now showing an increasing readiness to involve healers in their practices and hospitals.

In general, healing is about as natural and non-invasive as you can get and there is absolutely no evidence it can do anyone the slightest harm (except to your wallet, though many healers don't charge). So the moral is, if you feel drawn to it give it a try. Find someone with a good reputation, preferably in treating back pain sufferers, and see what happens. It might just work.

Homoeopathy

Homoeopathy is a complete system of medicine originating more than 200 years ago with a German doctor named Samuel Hahnemann (although the ancient Greeks already had similar ideas). The scientific world is still in dispute about how it works but there seems little doubt it does work from the evidence not only of successfully treated patients but a string of clinical studies going back many years.

Homoeopathy is based on the principle Hahnemann put forward, after experimenting on himself, that 'like cures like'. Homoeopathy means 'similar suffering' and homoeopaths believe the cure for a particular illness lies in giving the patient a remedy whose effects mimic his or her symptoms. So, for example, someone with muscular strain could be given a tiny dose of the remedy *arnica* (mountain daisy) which causes bruising in the belief it will draw out or trigger the patient's own natural·healing process.

Medical versus non-medical homoeopaths

If you want homoeopathy your doctor is likely to recommend you see a homoeopathic *doctor* rather than a homoeopath without conventional medical training. This is mainly because many doctors are sceptical of the skills of non-medical therapists and warn against them (non-medical or 'lay' homoeopaths usually prefer to call themselves 'professional homoeopaths'). Basically the choice is yours but if you are agonizing over it the following guidelines may help:

- A doctor can work within the state health service, so for those countries, such as Britain, with a free service using a doctor means you can get free treatment.
- A doctor has direct access to any amount of medical tests or other parts of the state health service you may need.
- A professional homoeopath is a specialist in the subject and frequently knows a great deal more about the range of remedies available (called the 'materia medica') and the symptoms they are used to treat (called the 'repertory') than most doctors who only study homoeopathy as an addition to their medical training and not for the same length of time.
- Homoeopathic remedies are the only working tools a pro-fessional homoeopath has (they have no drugs to fall back on if they fail) so their diagnostic and observational skills have to be highly developed.

The best guidance is, if you feel reassured by the fact that your practitioner is a doctor stick with a doctor. Back pain is not an obvious problem to see any kind of homoeopath about so it might be better to see a *recommended* profes-sional homoeopath for whom 'thinking homoeopathically' with flair and imagination is second nature. Alternatively call one of the homoeopathic organizations (Appendix A) for advice and further information.

Symptoms, seen from the homoeopath's viewpoint, are good indicators of how your body is trying to bring about healing. If they are progressing in a good direction nature will be left to do its own work. If your body seems to be going round in circles trying to sort out your back, for example, and has got stuck in the process the homoeopath will try to match your *symptom picture* to a suitable *remedy picture*.

This means working out which naturally occurring substance would produce the very symptoms you now have if it were given to a symptom-free person in irritating enough ('toxic') doses. This method of prescribing is the basic homoeopathic principle and is called the 'Law of Similars'. You will be given a remedy which will nudge you gently in the direction your body is already travelling.

The main problem with homoeopathy is that it is only as good as the person practising it, because there are so many remedies for the same condition and the right one has to be found for *you*. It takes years of dedicated training and practice to become good at it, and can't really be tagged on to conventional training as an afterthought. Yet many doctors have trained in homoeopathy and enjoy using it because it *is* so safe, gentle and effective.

Magnetotherapy

Magnetotherapy is simply the use of magnets to promote and reinforce the healing process. The therapy follows very much the principles behind acupuncture. Small magnets are applied to specific parts of the body or a magnetic current is directed on to the body and this encourages muscles to relax and blood to flow, so reducing inflammation and increasing regeneration. Therapists tend to use one of two methods to deliver the magnetic field:

- The static, or fixed, field method (usually using magnets sewn into a strap or belt or inserted into special plasters and applied to the affected area).
- The 'pulsed', or alternating, field method. (A special machine sends out a magnetic field generated electrically. The field is turned up and down to apply the field at regular intervals.)

Practitioners are divided between which is the better method but there is now plenty of research to show that both are extremely effective in helping problems of back pain, especially where there is muscle spasm. There is also good evidence that magnet therapy helps other treatments, particularly acupuncture and manipulation, to last.

Specific problems of back pain helped by magnetotherapy are sciatica, lumbago, joint pain, neck and shoulder pain, torticollis, whiplash and rheumatic pain. It also helps in cases of severe bruising, tendinitis and fibrositis and is said to accelerate the repair of broken bones.

Reflexology

Reflexology is simply described as foot massage but this does not really explain it enough. Reflexology is a modern revival of a healing method believed to have been widely practised in the ancient world with probable links with acupuncture and acupressure.

Like both acupuncture and acupressure, reflexology is based on the idea that lines of energy run through the body and these lines link all the major organs to specific 'reflex' points in the feet. According to reflexologists the bottom of each foot can be 'mapped' with areas or 'zones' which correspond to these various organs (*see figure 9*) and the organs can be affected by putting the reflex points under pressure.

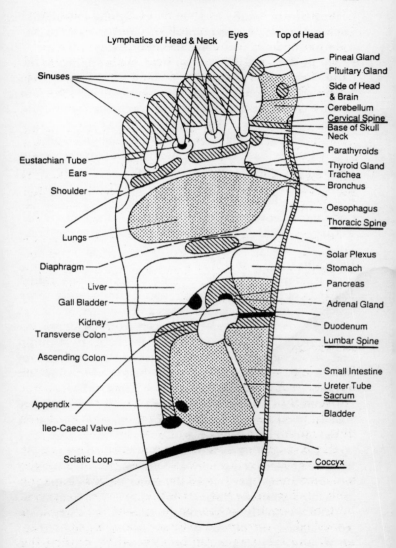

Fig 9. Reflexology 'zones' on the right foot

Pressure is usually applied by using the thumb and fingers. No pain means no problem – but any sort of discomfort or pain is said to indicate a problem in the corresponding area of the body and pressure is applied to the painful point. Sometimes this is distinctly uncomfortable but by working on the point for a few moments the pain usually eases and a response may occur in the affected organ.

So a headache might be relieved by having pressure applied to the base of the big toe (which corresponds to the base of the neck) and back pain by pressing along the arch of the foot (which looks like the curve of the spine). But even without this direct link to specific parts of the body most people testify to the fact that the therapy has a strong relaxing effect. In this way it will improve circulation and benefit most bodily functions whether it helps individual organs or not.

A modern 'high-tech' version of reflexology called *Vacuflex*, which claims to achieve better results more quickly by using special felt boots and a system of suction pads, has recently been introduced from Denmark via South Africa. Air is drawn out of the boots by a pump and the feet given an 'all-over' squeeze from the vacuum that results. The suction pads are then used to stimulate various reflex points on the feet, legs, arms and hands.

Though still in its infancy, early results with studies on back pain using Vacuflex look promising. One reason is thought to be that the bladder 'meridian' is very easy to access using this method and it is the bladder meridian that governs the muscles and other tissues running up and down either side of the spine – so often the culprits in maintaining chronic back pain.

This therapy is suggested for people for whom even good 'hands-on' therapy does not appear to 'hold' (last) or who are either particularly sensitive to, or do not respond to, any treatment at all.

Summary

Energy therapies undoubtedly have their place in the treatment of back pain but at what point you decide to try one will be a matter of what improvement you are getting so far, and your level of patience.

Therapies that treat your immediate physical symptoms are obviously most people's first thought and there is no doubt that some psychological therapies can also help in relaxing tissues and easing some of the mental and emotional pressures behind them. But if neither of these are getting you anywhere, energy therapies are your next step.

Discuss your problem with your present practitioner, to see whether a break from the treatment is due, and he may well be able to suggest someone in the field of 'energy-balancing therapies' who could help (or see Chapter 10 'How to find and choose a natural therapist'). You may, like many people, find some of them a bit far-fetched but the evidence that they help is there and if you do have a grumbling health problem which you think might be holding back the healing process in your back, or your back just isn't improving, keep an open mind until you've given them a try.

How to find and choose a natural therapist

Tips and guidelines for finding reliable help

We no longer (quite) live in the days when practitioners like herbalists were thought to be witches and were regularly burnt or drowned – though even in these 'enlightened' times many natural therapists are still persecuted for their beliefs by those with uncertain motives. It is now much easier to find a good therapist.

The main problem facing would-be patients is not only the sheer variety but the lack of organization in many therapies in most countries. The very explosion in their popularity has been at the root of this in most cases but it has resulted in a confusion that leaves many people wondering who to go to for what and where. Most important of all, perhaps, it has left the all-important question of who can they trust and rely on hanging in the air.

In most Western countries natural therapists are now busy trying to set up regulatory bodies to overcome this confusion and give the public some peace of mind. Some, such as chiropractors and osteopaths, have very largely got there – but many still have a way to go and others may never get there. In this situation what is the seeker after healing to do?

Beginning the search

Natural therapies have existed for as long as human beings have lived on earth, and finding a good practitioner has been and is a matter of tuning in to the community 'bush telegraph'. Word of mouth is still the best way of finding the right practitioner.

Speak to anyone whose opinion you respect, especially if they have had a back problem treated successfully by a natural therapist. (You will also want to know who to avoid.)

What other ways can you try? There are several.

Doctors' surgeries

If you need to be seen quickly and you don't have time for this process try your local doctor. Doctors' attitudes do vary (see Chapter 6) so be prepared to hear anything from a dire warning to a strong recommendation.

Natural health centres

Your nearest natural health centre should be happy to advise you. Your first impressions will often be a good guide to the quality of service they provide. For example, are the staff friendly and well informed? Is the place clean and comfortable? Does the atmosphere help you to feel better from the moment you walk in? It should. It matters. You are bringing them your trust and your custom, and both should be treated with the utmost respect.

The natural health clinic may have useful leaflets explaining the therapies and introducing the practitioners. In a well-run practice, the receptionist or owner will be well versed in the uses of different therapies too.

You may still be unsure after your first impressions whether to book in or not. If you are not happy to take the advice of an unqualified clinic owner or receptionist this is fair enough, and not uncommon. So ask to meet the person who might be treating you, just to test the waters. Even eye contact and a handshake are a good start, and this should be possible, even in a busy practice.

This is not the moment to tell your whole life history but some practices do offer you the chance to do that in a free consultation (usually 15 minutes) just to see whether you have come to the right place or not.

Local practitioners

You can also contact a local practitioner of a therapy other than the one you are looking for, to recommend a person in the field you want. Practitioners tend to know who's who in the area, and should be happy to help out. The same goes for any practitioner you might know socially, and therefore may not wish to consult, but who should be able to help you find the right person.

Healthfood stores and alternative bookshops

The staff in these kinds of shops often have good 'local knowledge' as well as an interest in the subject of natural therapies. The shop may well have a pinboard with local practitioners' business cards on it. Remember, though, the most experienced and well-established practitioners do not need this kind of advertising, so you might miss out on them altogether if you don't actually check up by asking.

Other sources of local knowledge

Don't forget your local pharmacist who may be just the person you are looking for as a link between conventional medicine and natural therapists.

The local library or information office may be another good source of contact, especially for finding self-help groups. Such groups can be useful because they consist of lay people who have already tried and tested various therapies and therapists. Bear in mind, though, that they are also often the people with very hard-to-shift pain so prepare yourself for some negative opinion too.

Computers (using a 'modem') can be good sources of information and others worth trying are health farms, beauty therapists, and citizens' advice bureaux.

If you draw a blank

You may need to find a less direct way to your natural therapist than by word of mouth but this need not be a problem. If you follow all the advice below you will still have checked them out thoroughly by the time you come to visit them.

'Umbrella' organizations

If you cannot find anyone by word of mouth, or if you want to know more about a therapist's qualifications, contact the national umbrella organizations for the nat-ural therapies (they are listed in Appendix A). They have lists of practitioners that amount to official registers in the case of the bigger therapies with their own regula-tory bodies already in place.

It is better to phone than to write because this will itself give you a pretty good idea of how well organized and 'switched on' the organizations are. When you phone you may find that the therapy you are asking about has several different associations. A small charge may be made for each organization's register but if you can afford it get the lot and make up your own mind.

Newspapers, magazines and local directories

Many therapists do now advertise in local directories, partly for ease of reference and partly to keep their name in the public eye. If you find someone local in this way it's a good idea to talk to them and check them out first.

Ten ways of finding a therapist

- word of mouth (usually the best method)
- your local family medical centres
- your local natural health centres
- your local healthfood shops
- health farms and beauty treatment centres
- local patient support groups
- national therapy organizations (but see below)
- computer networks (you need a 'modem')
- public libraries and information centres
- local directories, newspapers and magazines

Checking professional organizations

Some organizations are genuine groups that really keep a check on their members, while others seem to spring up like weeds in order to collect membership fees and give themselves credibility. This section helps you do your own weeding.

Why do professional organizations exist?

The purposes of governing bodies for natural therapies are:

- to keep up-to-date lists of their members so you can check whether someone really is on their list or not
- to protect you by making sure that their members are fully trained, licensed and insured against accident, negligence and malpractice
- to give you someone to complain to if you are unhappy with any aspect of treatment you have received, and you feel you can't sort the matter out with your therapist directly
- to protect their members by giving good ethical and legal advice

- to represent their members when laws which might affect them are being made
- to work towards improvements in education for their members, both before and after qualifying
- to work towards greater awareness of the benefit of each therapy in conventional medical circles
- to improve public awareness of the benefit of each therapy.

Questions to ask of professional organizations

The points listed above are observed to the letter by some organizations, and are totally ignored by others. A good organization will publish clear and simple information on its status and purposes along with its membership list but few seem to do this. You may need to contact them again on receiving your list and ask the following questions.

- When was the association founded? (You may be reassured by some that have been around for 50 years or more while others are brand new. If the association is new, however, don't reject it out of hand: ask why it was formed. It may be innovative.)
- How many members does it have? (Size reflects public demand, on the basis that not many therapists could survive in that therapy if there was no call for it. The bigger organizations generally have a better track record and greater public acceptance. Smaller associations may just reflect the fact that the therapy is very specialized or still in its infancy, though, and this is not necessarily a bad thing.)
- When was the *therapy* it represents started? (Some are as old as time and others are the latest innovations, often lacking in research or experienced practitioners. If you are not happy to be a guinea-pig leave the pioneering to others.)

- Is it a charity or educational trust – with a proper con-stitution, management committee and published accounts – or is it a private limited company? (Charities have to be non-profit making, working in the public interest, and open to inspection at any time. Private companies don't.)
- Is it part of a larger network of organizations? (If so this implies that it is interested in progress by consen-sus with other groups, not just in furthering its own aims. By and large groups that go their own way are more suspect than those who 'join in'.)
- Does the organization have a code of ethics (uphold-ing standards of professional behaviour) and discipli-nary procedures? (If so, what are they?)
- How do their members gain admission to their regis-ter? Is it linked to only one school? (Beware of associa-tions whose heads are also head of the school they represent: unbiased help may be in short supply when you most need it with this type of 'one man band'.)
- Do members have to have proof of professional indemnity insurance? This should cover:
  – accidental damage to yourself or your property while you are on the practitioner's work premises
  – negligence (the failure of the practitioner to exercise the 'duty of care' owed to you, or his falling below the standard of clinical competence demanded by his qualifications, either of these resulting in an overall worsening of your problem)
  – malpractice (a 'falling from grace' over professional conduct. It could involve dishonesty, breach of confi-dentiality – your personal details should *never* be dis-cussed with a third person without your permission – or sexual misconduct.)

Checking training and qualifications

If you have reassured yourself so far but are still puzzled by what the training actually involves, ask a few more questions.

- How long is the training?
- Is it full or part time?
- If it is part time but longer than a full-time course leading to the same qualification, does the time spent at lectures and in clinic add up to the same as a full-time course overall? (In other words, is it a short-cut?)
- Does it include seeing patients under supervision at a college clinic and in real practices?
- What do the initials after the therapist's name mean? (Some therapists seem to join every organization under the sun, just to have lots of impressive-looking letters after their names, while others really have studied two or three therapies in great depth.)
- Are the qualifications recognized? If so, by whom? (This is becoming more relevant as the therapy organizations group together and start to form state-recognized registers in many countries. But the really important thing is if the qualifications are recognized by an independent outside assessment authority.)

Making the choice

Making the final choice is a matter of using a combination of common sense and intuition and giving someone a try. Don't forget that the most important part of the whole healing process is your resolve to get better. The next most important part is that you feel comfortable with your chosen therapist.

One practical point with a painful back is getting to and from the therapist's workplace. Many people think that the best practitioners must be in big cities and make

The British Medical Association's opinion

In its long-awaited second report into the practice of natural medicine in Britain, published in June 1993, the British Medical Association recommended that anyone seeking the help of a non-conventional therapist – doctor or patient – should ask the following questions:

- Is the therapist registered with a professional organization?
- Does the professional organization have
  — a public register?
  — a code of practice?
  — an effective disciplinary procedure and sanction?
  — a complaints mechanism?
- What qualification does the therapist hold?
- What training was involved in getting the qualification(s)?
- How many years has the therapist been practising?
- Is the therapist covered by professional indemnity insurance?

The BMA said that although it would like to see natural therapies regulated by law, with a single regulating body for each therapy, it did not think that all therapies needed regulating. For the majority, it said, 'the adoption of a code of practice, training structures and voluntary registration would be sufficient'.

Complementary Medicine: New Approaches to Good Practice (Oxford University Press, 1993)

great efforts to cover long distances to see the 'top person'. But when you have a back problem you don't want to arrive in howling pain from your journey there, and upset the good effects of treatment on your journey back. So do not hesitate to choose someone local if you can, at least first off.

(If your problem does need the attention of a 'top person' the practitioner should be able to refer you reliably 'up the ladder' to someone more suitable in any case.

The advantage of this approach is that your existing therapist will be able to supply a record of your treatments so far – and in difficult cases two heads are often better than one.)

What it is like seeing a natural therapist

In a word, different. But it is also very natural. Since most therapists, even in those countries with state health systems, still work mainly privately there is no established uniform or common outlook. Although they may all share more or less a belief in the principles outlined in Chapter 6 you are liable to come across individuals as different as chalk from cheese, representing all walks of life, from the rich to the poor, the politically left to the politically right. That means you will come across as much variety in dress, thinking and behaviour as there are fashions, from the elegant and formal to the positively informal and 'woolly-haired' (though, for image reasons, many now wear a white coat to look more like a doctor!).

Equally, you will find their premises very different – reflecting their attitudes to their work and the world. Some will present a 'brass plaque' image, working in a clinic or room away from home with a receptionist and brisk efficiency, while others will see you in their living room surrounded by pot plants and domestic clutter. Remember, though, image may be some indication of status but it is little guarantee of ability. You are as likely to find a therapist of quality working from home as one in a formal clinic.

There are some characteristics, however, probably the most important ones, you will find common to all natural therapists. They will:

● give you far more time than you are used to with a family doctor. An initial consultation will rarely last less than an hour, and often longer. During it they will ask you all about yourself so they can form a proper understanding of what makes you tick and what may be the fundamental cause(s) of your problem.

- charge you for their time and for any remedies they prescribe, which they may well sell you themselves from their own stocks. But many therapists offer reduced fees, and even waive fees altogether, for deserving cases or for people who genuinely cannot afford it.

Sensible precautions

- Be sceptical of anyone who 'guarantees' you a cure. No one (not even doctors) can.
- Query any attempt to book you in for a 'course of treatments' for back pain. No one can predict from the first visit how soon you will be better. In any case you may only need a case history taken, examination and very little treatment (if that) to see how sensitive you are to treatment. You may be asked to book in for two or three sessions ahead, though, if it is a busy practice. This ensures that you have treatments at the right intervals for you. You should be able to cancel without penalty any sessions which prove unnecessary.
- Although most practitioners practise for fees no ethical person will ask for fees in advance of treatment unless for special tests or medicines, but even this is unusual. If you are asked for 'down payments' of any sort ask exactly what for and if you don't like the reasons refuse to pay.
- Be wary if you are not asked about any medication you are on (but try to be specific if you are asked: the colour of pills is not much for the therapist to go on!) – and be especially wary if the therapist tells you to stop suddenly any medically-prescribed drug, particularly any you have been on long-term. In general it is easier

for natural therapists to treat you 'in the clear' rather than through a haze of painkillers, so they are always likely to steer you away from drugs if they can, but consult your doctor first. (In the case of back pain, though, this does not include short-term painkillers you may have been told to use 'as needed'.) A responsible therapist should be happy to contact your doctor to discuss your drugs (and a responsible doctor should be happy to discuss them with the therapist).

- Note the quality of the therapist's touch when you go for manual therapy for back pain. The therapist's touch should be firm and professional yet gentle and sensitive at all times. It may be delicate on occasions but it should always be purposeful. It should *never*, *ever* be lingering or suggestive. The purpose of hand contact around the breast area or genitals should always be explained and your permission should always be sought beforehand. Although it may seem very intimate the practitioner would not be doing their job if they didn't, say, check for a hernia in your groin or feel for the alignment of your pubic bone sometimes. If you have back pain in the chest area the rib movement at the front may need to be examined and breasts do get in the way!

- If the practitioner is of the opposite sex you are entitled to have someone of your choice in the room at the same time. Be immediately suspicious if this is not allowed. No ethical therapist will refuse this sort of request, and if they do it is probably best to have nothing more to do with them.

What to do if you don't get better

If you have had a few sessions and all is well except that you really are no better try talking to your practitioner about how you feel (see also Chapter 6 'If at first you don't succeed'). Ideally an alert practitioner should notice your disappointment and bring the subject up first. Consider first, though, that various things might be holding you back. For example, impatience. Solving the puzzle of a painful back is not like hitting it with a drug. It may just need more patience on both sides. If you have been suffering for a long time you may be doubly keen to get the problem sorted out. But remember you are completely new to the therapist, who needs to get to know you, your problem and your lifestyle. Even so, after three or four sessions you should have made at least *some* noticeable progress in terms of pain, mobility or general well-being, and if not you should have a clear explanation from the therapist as to why it will take longer. The problem could be one of the following.

- *Sabotage* You might be doing something that aggravates your condition, for example sleeping on your front when you have a neck problem.
- *Resistance to co-operating fully* You might be reluctant to give up some favourite sport so have convinced yourself that you don't need to mention, for example, the bungee-jumping!
- *Wrong frequency of treatment* Your back might not be having time to 'settle' between treatments and this can sometimes 'stir things up' for a few days. On the other hand, you might not be having enough treatments, particularly if you have an old problem of, say, stiffness. If the cost of having more frequent treatments is a problem suggest having more frequent but shorter treatments at a lower price if possible.
- *Wrong diagnosis* Getting it wrong is not difficult with a problem with as many different causes as back pain. The therapist may suggest getting a second opinion.
- *Wrong practitioner, right therapy* If the therapy is what you want but you cannot relax with the practitioner for some reason, change therapists.

- *Wrong therapy* You may be unsuitable for the therapy you have chosen. You may be too mobile, too sensitive, deeply depressed or lacking in vital energy. But don't give up. Keep searching for an answer: sometimes this comes from outside and sometimes from within.
- *Additional therapy is needed to support treatment* This follows on from the last point. Ask your existing practitioner for advice.

What to do if things go wrong

A practitioner is in a position of trust, and is charged with a 'duty of care' to you at all times. This does not mean you are entitled to a 'cure' just because you've paid for treatment. But if you feel you are being treated unfairly, incompetently or unethically you have several options.

- Tackle the matter at the source of the problem, with your practitioner, either verbally or in writing.
- If he or she works in a place like a clinic, health farm or sports centre tell the management. They also have a duty to protect the public and should treat complaints fairly and discreetly.
- Contact the practitioner's professional organization. They should have an independent panel which investigates complaints fully and disciplines its members.
- If the offence committed is a criminal one report it to the police (but be prepared for the problem of proving one person's word against another's).
- If you feel compensation is due to you see a solicitor for advice.

Short of a public court case, the worst thing for a truly incompetent or unethical practitioner is bad publicity. Tell everybody about your experiences. People only need to hear the same sort of comments from a few different sources and that practitioner will sink without trace. Before you do it, though, try the other measures open to you first and give yourself time to consider things calmly. Vengeance is not really healing.

A word of warning Don't make malicious allegations without substance. Such actions are themselves a criminal offence and could get you in deeper trouble than the trouble you hope for the practitioner.

Summary

This book has been a short introduction to two huge subjects – back pain and the safest, gentlest and most effective way out of it. Almost every therapy has ways of trying to help people with back pain. This is because so many people suffer with it, and it touches those who witness their suffering.

People who become natural therapists are rarely in it just for the money. It often takes years to train and it always takes years to build up a successful practice. Many natural therapists started just like you, in search of a solution to their problem which no one in the world of conventional medicine had been able to sort out. They were often helped beyond their wildest dreams.

It is experiences like these that give natural therapists the courage of their convictions in therapies that have been ridiculed too often in the past by people who should have known better. But times are changing – at last – and you are part of that change.

So, take courage. Take responsibility for your back and the way it is now and do what you can for yourself. In the future, if you still need help, go and see a natural therapist. Your back may never look back!

Glossary

Acute Short-lived symptoms that start suddenly.

Arthritis Joint pain from disease or injury.

Cartilage Protective covering for bones where they make joints.

Chronic Long-term and persistently recurring symptoms that start gradually.

Connective tissue The 'packaging material' of the body that gathers together to make tendons, ligaments and cartilage.

Discs Tough-walled but soft-centred 'shock absorbers' between the vertebrae.

Facet joints Chain of small joints down each side of the spine.

Fascia Sheets of connective tissue that separate sections of the body and form coverings for all its structures.

Fibrositis Muscle pain

Inflammation The body's first response to injury, with redness, swelling, heat and pain.

Ligaments Tough bands of connective tissue that stabilize joints.

Lumbago Low backache.

Lymphatic system The body's 'drainage' system and an important part of the immune system.

Muscle Bundles of elastic fibres that can contract and cause movement.

Rheumatism Pain in joints or muscles not caused by infection or obvious injury.

Sacro-iliac joints Joints either side of the buttock crease that join the base of the spine to the pelvis.

Sciatica Pain running down the back of the leg.

Tendon Tough band of connective tissue joining muscle to bone.

Trauma The medical word for injury.

Vertebra A single bone of the spine (plural *vertebrae*).

APPENDIX A

Useful organizations

The following listing of organizations is for information only and does not imply any endorsement, nor do the organizations listed necessarily agree with the views expressed in this book.

INTERNATIONAL

International Federation of Practitioners of Natural Therapeutics
46 Pulens Crescent
Sheet
Petersfield
Hampshire GU31 4DH, UK.
Tel 01730 266790
Fax 01730 260058

AUSTRALASIA

Acupuncture Ethics and Standards Organization
PO Box 84
Merrylands
New South Wales 2160
Australia.

Australian Council on Chiropractic and Osteopathic Education
941 Nepean Highway
Mornington
Victoria 3931
Australia.

Australian Natural Therapists Association
PO Box 308
Melrose Park
South Australia 5039.
Tel 8297 9533
Fax 8297 0003

Australian Traditional Medicine Society
PO Box 442 *or*
Suite 3, First Floor,
120 Blaxland Road
Ryde
New South Wales 2112
Australia.
Tel 2808 2825
Fax 2809 7570

New Zealand Natural Health Practitioners Accreditation Board
PO Box 37-491
Auckland, New Zealand.
Tel 9 625 9966
Supported by 15 therapy organizations.

New Zealand Register of Acupuncturists
PO Box 9950
Wellington 1
New Zealand.

New Zealand Register of Osteopaths
PO Box 11 – 853
Wellington 1
New Zealand.

NORTH AMERICA

American Academy of Medical Preventics
6151 West Century Boulevard,
Suite 1114
Los Angeles
California 90045, USA.
Tel 213 645 5350

American Academy of Osteopathy
1127 Mount Vernon Road
PO Box 750
Newark
Ohio 43058 – 0750
USA.

American Association of Acupuncture and Oriental Medicine
National Acupuncture
Headquarters
1424 16th Street NW, Suite 501
Washington DC 20036,
USA.

American Association of Naturopathic Physicians
2800 East Madison Street, Suite 200
Seattle
Washington 98112, USA
or
PO Box 20386
Seattle
Washington 98102, USA.
Tel 206 323 7610
Fax 206 323 7612

American Holistic Medical Association
4101 Lake Boone Trail, Suite 201
Raleigh
North Carolina 27607, USA.
Tel 919 787 5146
Fax 919 787 4916

American Institute of Homoeopathy
1500 Massachusetts Avenue NW
Washington DC 20005
USA.

American Osteopathic Association
142 East Ohio Street
Chicago
Illinois 60611
USA.
Tel 312 280 5800

B.K.S. Iyengar Yoga National Association of the United States
8223 West Third Street
Los Angeles
California 90038,
USA.

North American Society of Homoeopaths
4712 Aldrich Avenue
Minneapolis 55409,
USA.

Canadian Holistic Medical Association
700 Bay Street
PO Box 101, Suite 604
Toronto
Ontario M5G 1Z6, Canada.
Tel 416 599 0447

SOUTHERN AFRICA

South African Homoeopaths, Chiropractors & Allied Professions Board
PO Box 17055
0027 Gooenkloof
South Africa
Tel 2712 466 455

UNITED KINGDOM

British Association for Counselling
1 Regent Place
Rugby
Warwickshire CV21 2PJ.
Tel 01788 578328

British Chiropractic Association
29 Whitley Street
Reading
Berks RG2 0EG.
Tel 01734 757557
Fax 01734 757257

British Complementary Medicine Association
St Charles Hospital
Exmoor Street
London W10 6DZ.
Tel 0181-964 1205
Fax 0181-964 1207

British Holistic Medical Association
Trust House
Royal Shrewsbury Hospital
South
Shrewsbury
Shropshire SY3 8XF.
Tel 01743 261155
Fax 01743 3536373

Council for Complementary & Alternative Medicine
179 Gloucester Place
London NW1 6DX.
Tel 0171-724 9103
Fax 0171-724 5330

Institute for Complementary Medicine
PO Box 194
London SE16 1QZ.
Tel 0171-237 5165
Fax 0171-237 5175

Health Education Authority
Hamilton House
Mabledon Place
London WC1H 9TX.
Tel 0171-383 3833
Fax 0171-387 0550

National Back Pain Association
16 Elmtree Road
Teddington
Middlesex TW11 8ST.
Tel 0181-977 5474

**Osteopathic Information
Service**
56 London Street
or
PO Box 2074
Reading
Berks RG1 4SQ
Tel 01734 512051

Yoga Therapy Centre
Royal London Homoeopathic
Hospital
60 Great Ormond Street
London WC1N 3HR
Tel 0171-833 7267
Fax 0171 833 7292

APPENDIX B

Useful further reading

Acupressure for Common Ailments, Chris Jarmey and John Tindall (Gaia Books, UK, 1991)

Acupuncture, George Lewith (Thorsons, UK, 1982)

Beating Back Pain, John Tanner (Dorling Kindersley, UK, 1987)

Book of Massage, Lucinda Lidell and others (Ebury Press, UK, 1984)

Conquering Pain, Sampson Lipton (Martin Dunitz, UK, 1984)

Family Guide to Alternative Medicine, ed Patrick Pietroni (The Reader's Digest Association, UK, 1991)

The Patient's Guide to Medical Tests, Cathey and Edward Pinckney (Facts on File Publications, USA, 1986)

Healers on Healing, ed Richard Carlson and Benjamin Shield (Jeremy P Tarcher, USA, 1989, and Rider/Century Hutchinson, UK, 1990)

Moon Over Water: Meditation for Beginners, Jessica Macbeth (Gateway Books, UK, 1991)

Nutritional Medicine, Stephen Davies and Alan Stewart (Pan Books, UK, 1987)

Raw Energy, Leslie and Susannah Kenton (Arrow Books, UK, 1989)

The Alexander Technique Workbook, Richard Brennan (Element, UK/USA, 1992)

The Alternative Health Guide, Brian Inglis and Ruth West (Michael Joseph, UK, 1983)

The Art of Reflexology, Inge Dougans and Suzanne Ellis (Element Books, UK/USA, 1992)

The Healthy Back Book, Elizabeth Sharp (Element Books, UK/USA, 1993)

The Family Guide to Homoeopathy, Andrew Lockie (Hamish Hamilton, UK, 1990)

The New Holistic Herbal, David Hoffman (Element Books, UK/USA, 1990)

Yoga for Common Ailments, R Nagarathana, H R Nagendra, Robin Monro (Gaia Books, UK, 1990)

Index

abdominal muscles, to
   strengthen 58–9
accidents, damage from 36–7
acupressure 116–17
acupuncture 114–16
acute conditions 24
Alexander Technique 90–91
aortic aneurism 29
applied kinesiology, *see*
   kinesiology

Bach remedies 110
backs – people at risk of injury
   to 7–8;
   function of 10;
   composition of 10–14, 16–17;
   curves of 15;
   how it moves 15–17.
   See also pain; preventative
   measures; symptoms
backswing 47
baths 53
bed rest 32, 45–6
blood tests 67
bones, damage to 40–1
brain haemorrhage 31
British Medical Association
   (BMA) 81, 82, 85

chemonucleolysis 78
chiropody 71
chiropractic 82, 92–3
chronic conditions 24
circulatory system 18–19
coccyx 37
corsets *see* spinal supports

counselling 106–7
cranial osteopathy 41, 96–7
CT (CAT) scan 74

dentistry 71
dieting 55–7
discs 4, 14–15, 37–8
disease 6–7
doctors 63–4, 84–5
drugs 65–6, 137

electrocardiograph (ECG) 113
electromyography 75
endorphins 27
epidural injections 77
exercise 18, 54–5, 56–7, 58–61

fever 32
first aid for sore backs 45–53
fish oil 49–50
flower remedies 110–11
flu 32

'gate theory' 28
gallbladder problems 34
gynaecological problems 35

healers 117–19
healthfood stores 128
heart attack 29–30
herbs 50
homoeopathic remedies 50–1
homoeopathy 119–21
hot packs 52
hydrotherapy 51–3, 70
hypnotherapy 107

ice packs 51–2
injections 76–8
interferential therapy 69

joints 13, 15–17, 40

kidney problems 35–6
kinesiology, applied 58, 91–2

life force, concept of 113
lumbago 3
lung infections 32

magnetotherapy 121–2
Maitlands Mobilization 69
massage 38, 93–5
meditation 62, 108
meningitis 31
moxibustion 114
MRI scan 74
muscles 17, 41
myelogram 75

natural health centres 127–8
natural therapies – general
    principles 85–8; cost 97;
    self-checks with 137–9
natural therapists – general
    characteristics 135–6; checks
    on 136–7; complaints
    procedures 139–40
nerves 17, 39–40
neurology 73
NSAIDS 49

orthopaedics 73
orthotics 71
osteopathy 95–7
osteophytes 42
osteoporosis 42

pain – types of 3–6, 22–4;
    causes of 6–9, 20–1, 22–6,
    29–43; how it works 21–2;
    psychology of 26, 101–5;
    relief 27, 28, 49–50;
    threshold 27; clinics 72
pancreatitis 33
pelvis 13–14
physiotherapy 68–9
podiatry 71–2
posture 24–5, 100–101
preventive measures 44–62
professional organizations 129,
    130–32
psychotherapy 106

radiating pain 22–3
radiculography see myelogram
referred pain 22, 29
reflexology 122–4
rehabilitation centres 72, 79
relaxation 61–2, 108–10
rheumatoid arthritis 42–3, 49,
    72
rheumatology 72
rubs and sprays 53

sacro-cranial therapy 96–7
scans 74–5
scar tissue 38, 39, 46
sciatica 3, 39
sclerosant injections 77
shiatsu 116, 117
short wave diathermy 69
spinal deformities 41
spinal injuries 36–41
spinal supports 48–9
spondylitis 42, 43, 67
spondylosis 13, 42
steroid injections 39, 76–7
surgery 39, 73, 78–80, 83
symptoms of back problems 29,
    30–1, 32–43

TENS machines 70
tissue 6, 19; *see also* scar tissue
traction 47–8, 71
Traditional Chinese Medicine
    115–16

ulcers 32–3
ultrasound 69, 75

Vacuflex 124
vertebrae 10–13;
    crush fracture of 36–7
weight loss 55–7
whiplash 39

x-rays 67–8

yoga 62, 97–9

BHMA TAPES FOR HEALTH

*Practical self-help packages designed by
experts to make taking care of yourself easier*

Imagery For Relaxation by Duncan Johnson
Exercises in visualization to help relaxation and influence the functions
of the body and mind. To provide yourself with the opportunity to
learn more about your attitudes and neglected needs. To harness the
forces of the creative mind and change negative attitudes to life.

Getting To Sleep by Ashley Conway
A practical help with insomnia. Promotes relaxation and positive
thinking to put you in touch with your body's 'normal' sleep pattern.

Introduction To Meditation by Dr Sarah Eagger
This tape is a progressive learning programme of meditation exercises.
Teaching you how to begin using meditation for increasing your peace
of mind and well-being.

Coping With Persistent Pain by Dr James Hawkins
Teaches relaxation skills in a greater depth, and how to apply those
skills as a coping method during daily activities. To help promote
some form of normality into a life of constant pain.

Coping With Stress by Dr David Peters
A programme to teach you how to build the relaxation response into
your life. Understanding stress and dealing with it through relaxation
techniques.

The Breath Of Life by Dr Patrick Pietroni
A muscular relaxation technique which explores the connection
between stress and our breathing rhythm. With exercises on how to
control breathing to alleviate symptoms of stress.

Please write to the British Holistic Medical Association at Rowland
Thomas House, Royal Shrewbury Hospital South, Shrewsbury,
Shropshire, SY3 8XF for full details of tapes and mail order service.